GIB'S ODYSSEY

GIB'S ODYSSEY

One Man's Battle Against the Ravages of Lou Gehrig's

Disease and his Courageous Final Voyage

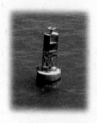

WALTER G. BRADLEY

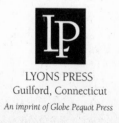

LYONS PRESS
Guilford, Connecticut
An imprint of Globe Pequot Press

Lyons Press is an imprint of Globe Pequot Press.

Text design: Elizabeth Kingsbury
Layout artist: Melissa Evarts
Project editor: Kristen Mellitt
Endpaper maps by Trailhead Graphics, Inc. © Morris Book
Publishing, LLC

Library of Congress Cataloging-in-Publication Data is available
on file.

ISBN 978-0-7627-7987-9
Printed in the United States of America

10 9 8 7 6 5 4 3 2 1

This book is dedicated to the millions of people who have died of amyotrophic lateral sclerosis (Lou Gehrig's disease), and the tens of thousands who will die every year until we find what causes ALS and how to prevent it.

Up-end the glass! New life is on the way.

Gib Peters

From: Gib Peters
To: All my family and friends
Subject: Why do I do this?

Marcia kissed me goodbye, Bill Schwessinger and Calvin ceremoniously tossed off the lines, and I eased my vessel off the seawall. It was May 19, 2004, at 10:30 a.m. And so it began. An odyssey to somewhere—maybe the Bahamas, New York, the Great Lakes, then down the Mississippi to the Gulf, or maybe none of these. If my boat and I hold together, maybe all of these and more.

The sky is clear light blue this morning and dotted with tiny puffs of cottony clouds. The air is calm and the heat is already building. It's the first summerlike day we've seen this year in Key West after an unusually windy, skuzzy spring. I set the throttles back and guide my boat east down the Riviera Canal to the Cow Key Channel, waving to the three shrinking figures on the seawall.

I find my way to the No. 1 marker at the southernmost end of Cow Key Channel and turn east, for New York, stopping at the Oceanside Marina for a fill-up of gas. At $2.37 a gallon today, and higher prices expected this summer, this is going to be one expensive dream. My twin Chevy V8s suck down gas like side-by-side porcelain toilets. But at least I'm finally under way.

And then it hits me. Is this really happening? Have I actually started this once-in-a-lifetime voyage?

Just before departure my good friend Jerry Cash turned to me and announced in a flash of understanding, "I know why you're doing this!" I mumbled an acknowledgment. He explained: "The adventure, the challenge, the time for reflection."

He was absolutely on the mark, of course. Jerry always is. But he couldn't have known the core inner reason for making a voyage, solo in a small vessel over such a distance. It wasn't entirely clear even to me until a few days after I left and perhaps still hasn't fully crystallized. But let me see if I can explain.

In February of 2003 I was diagnosed with Lou Gehrig's disease, or ALS. This is a progressive disease that in my case first showed its effects in weakness of the muscles of the tongue. Rather than beginning with weakness of the leg muscles and moving up, which is happening to a friend who has just contacted me, mine works from the top down and is called bulbar ALS. Two years ago my tongue just didn't want to move with the speed and accuracy that would produce effortless speech. For a lawyer, this is a serious impediment. As it spreads downwards, the arms, legs, and lungs stop working. But the disease, even in its final stages, leaves the mind sound and the senses alert. That's the really scary part for me.

Dr. Walter Bradley tells me that the process will extend for two or three years from the time of diagnosis. Toward the end, most of my body will be limp with paralysis, except my eyes and a few involuntary functions like the heart and digestive system. Unable to cough or breathe without ventilation support, my systems will fail. In the end I'll be "locked in," unable to move anything but my eyes. Somewhere along the line, he says I'll be unable to cough, will catch pneumonia, and die. He said it just like that. And I am glad he did because I know there's no doctor-dodging going on and I can plan the rest of my life.

Now, taking a cold, clinical look at all that, I've in some ways removed myself "from me" as though looking at a biological specimen in a petri dish—attentive to the progression and determined to figure out how much time this organism has left. It's an approach to living or dying that works for me. Otherwise, I would sink into a state of depression, sucking in all those around me and putting a sour exclamation point to the end of my life.

Overlaying the clinical picture is the inner need of a man to survive, to cope, to win. I'm no different. I'm determined to fight ALS every step of the way, but intellectually I know that I will lose the war. We are all fighting time, and sick or well, sooner or later, we will lose—but it's important to play the game full-tilt 'til the final buzzer. This just happens to be my clock that is running, and my moments that are precious. So this is how I choose to do it, and I am filled with unexplained contentment and peace.

Every good petri dish watcher has to have a way to tell if there has been change over time. So how do I measure the progression of my disease and project a curve against time into the future? Doc Bradley puts me through a series of strength tests every month or so. After sixteen months my tongue is all but paralyzed. Speech is difficult, if not impossible, and I've resorted to carrying a note-pad on a clipboard for personal communication. The phone is useless, but e-mailing is perfect for distant communication. My right arm has developed early signs of weakness. Ten months ago I could do thirteen reps with an eight-pound weight on the right, and fifteen on the left. Now I'm finding it difficult to lift the right arm at all. The left arm still works pretty well but is showing some signs of weakening. As I watch the movements in my petri dish, I see the left hand helping the right do its job more often now. On an emotional level it pisses me off more than it saddens me!

My legs are fine and able to carry me up the bridge ladder, forward to the ground tackle and around the aft deck of my boat. My neck muscles are weakening, and late in the day I am frequently unable to raise my chin off my chest. If I find myself walking down a long marina dock, I'll fake a thoughtful, left-hand-to-the-chin pose to keep my head up. That is what I call a victory! My neck brace is stored aboard somewhere, and I will get it out when I have to give up this ground too.

As simply as I can tell it, I want to provoke my ALS to a fight. A solo trek in a small boat provides the adventures, challenges, and solitude needed to test me. I want to beat it on every ground it chooses to challenge me and then reflect on which of us won the battle: the petri dish thing. I am calling it out for the fight of a lifetime. I won't let it just creep over me in my rocking chair back in Key West. I will try to outwit and out-manipulate it. This voyage is simply pure provocation of my disease and a way to face its devastation and brag about how I did it.

And I need to write. About who I am, how I lived, and how I challenged my death. I want my grands, great-grands, and the generations who come after them to know that I believe that it *is* about how you play the game.

Gib

Gib Peters was extraordinary, even before his illness developed and he set out on an odyssey that many an able-bodied person would find challenging.

A devoted husband and father of four. A successful banker, financial adviser, and newspaper columnist. A lawyer who never practiced his profession. A generous philanthropist, giving freely of his professional and personal time. A community activist. An accomplished sailor and airplane pilot. An electronics inventor and ham radio operator who was good with his hands. An academic administrator who quit his profession when about to become a college president, and took up a new career in business. An extrovert who liked to be alone with his own thoughts.

I first met Gib in June 2003. He was sixty-seven years old but looked ten years younger. He was an engaging, likable man, five feet ten inches tall, 210 pounds, and built like a tank. He had clearly been an athlete in his youth. His square ruddy face was handsome and his hair almost white. A wry smile played constantly around his lips. Gib wrote a humorous financial advice column for the local paper, the *Key West Citizen*. He was a great raconteur and hosted a weekly TV program. Gib was a larger-than-life personality in Key West, and his ALS was a topic of shocked public discussion.

He had been diagnosed with amyotrophic lateral sclerosis (ALS for short), or Lou Gehrig's disease, in March 2003. His reaction to this virtual death sentence was to decide to take on ALS and, if not beat it, at least give it a good fight. Gib's feeling was that he might not win the war, but he was certainly going to win a few battles along the way. He accomplished an extraordinary feat of endurance, far beyond the abilities of most of us. He gained some amazingly deep insights into life and death and shared these with friends, family, and, eventually, the world.

As Gib's disease progressed, his tongue weakened and his speech became unintelligible. He described his speech as being reduced to a "spit-mumble." He began having difficulty swallowing his saliva and would drool like a baby. His eating became slower, and he began to choke, first on liquids and later on solid food. He lost weight. I arranged for a tube to be put through his belly into his stomach. (We call this a PEG tube, for percutaneous endoscopic gastrostomy.) Gib was able to pour liquid nutrition into the tube, bypassing his throat to avoid choking and starvation.

This was Gib's condition when he first told me about his plan to pilot his twenty-nine-foot motor cruiser, the *Ka Ching*, single-handedly from his home in Key West, following the Intracoastal Waterway (ICW), to New York, the Great Lakes, and the Mississippi, making a great loop back to his home in Key West. For most healthy sixty-seven-year-olds, such a journey would be arduous, but I knew that the ALS was going to spread to Gib's spinal cord over the coming months and make it almost impossible for him to complete such a voyage.

Despite my insistence that his plans were unrealistic, Gib was obstinate and soon set off on what he called his own personal odyssey. ALS robbed him of the ability to speak by phone. So during his voyage he wrote e-mails to his family and friends that told of his experiences on the journey and his insights into the meaning of life and the inevitability of his own death. Terry Schmida, features editor at the *Key West Citizen*, invited Gib to publish this material in the newspaper. Gib accepted the invitation with these words: "My insufferable ego and a writer's addiction to having lots of readers have overcome my natural humbleness and strong inclination to decline." The result was a series of alternately heart-wrenching and hilarious weekly columns in the *Citizen*.

In 1996 Gib Peters had no idea of the fate that awaited him. He was strong, successful, and popular. He was beginning to have the time and money to indulge some of the dreams he had when he moved to Key West, one of which was to own a seagoing vessel.

He bought a small motorboat, a seventeen-foot Mako that he called *Off the Wall*, and took his family on many trips around the Keys. They often went west to the Marquesas and northeast to the Upper Keys. Boating, fishing, and scuba diving became passions of the whole family.

They loved to dive on the beautiful Florida reefs, especially those at John Pennekamp State Park, where some say the fish are more brilliant than those at the Australian Great Barrier Reef. John Pennekamp State Park is the dive capital of Florida and home to the underwater nine-foot bronze statue, *Christ of the Abyss*. In 1965 this gift of the Italian scuba manufacturer Egidi Cressi was placed in thirty feet of water near Dry Rocks Reef in the park and is a magnet for divers. It is a reproduction of the original *Il Cristo Degli Abissi,* which is mounted on the bottom of the Mediterranean in the Italian Riviera near Portofino.

Gib loved his Mako. When he came into the bank one Monday after a weekend working on the engine, one of his clients said there couldn't be anything wrong with a banker who had grease under his fingernails! He would take the boat out fishing in all weather and was often out there for eight or nine hours at a time. He liked to be alone to think. Friends like Bill Schwessinger, who knew the sea and its risks, worried about Gib. He would often stay out during storms when, in Bill's words, "any sensible man would have run for safe harbor. I told him he was taking too much of a risk, that man must respect the sea."

In 2000 Gib sold the *Off the Wall*, much to the relief of his friends. In its place he bought a twenty-nine-foot Wellcraft that was to become the love of his life, second only to his "bride," Marcia. The new boat was twenty years old and needed a lot of work. He would often ask his friend Dick Moody, who was good with mechanical things: "Will you just come over and look at this to see if I have gotten it right?" He spent all his free time working on the boat, which was docked behind his house on Riviera Canal. At times he became so engrossed in his projects that he seemed almost to forget that Marcia, his children, and his friends existed.

About the time that Gib bought the Wellcraft—three years before he was diagnosed with ALS—his personality seemed to change. He became more reclusive and did not want to talk to people. When Gib and Marcia went to a party, he would want to go home after an hour, while Marcia wanted to stay till the end as they had always done before. On many of these occasions, Gib would take the car home, and Bill and Anita Schwessinger would later give Marcia a ride home.

He drifted into day-trading stocks. He would closet himself with his computer and not surface for a whole day. Sometimes he would make $20,000 in a day, but at other times he would lose just as much. When Bill Schwessinger visited, all he could get out of Gib was a hello. Gib clearly wasn't feeling sociable.

Gib had been a long-term board member of the Mel Fisher Maritime Museum, involved in handling the treasure recovered from the wreck of the 1622 Spanish galleon, the *Nuestra Señora de Atocha*, off the Marquesas, west of Key West. In 2001, when he came into the dusty office of Madeleine Burnside, executive director of the museum, he complained, "Gosh, this room is full of mold!" It appeared that he had become allergic to molds, suffering frequent sinus infections. He went to the Mayo Clinic in Rochester, Minnesota, to try to find the cause of his allergies. Over the next eighteen months, they operated several times on his sinuses, all to no avail, except that he completely lost his sense of smell.

Whether the personality change and allergies had anything to do with his later development of ALS, I don't know. Some people with bulbar ALS have personality changes due to degeneration of the frontal parts of the brain, a condition called fronto-temporal dementia. But Gib's personality change began three years before he started to slur his speech, which would be very unusual, particularly since the personality change did not get worse with time.

A year before he knew he had ALS, Gib began to complain of fatigue, which is very common in ALS, though it does not usually come before other signs of the disease. Six months before he received the diagnosis of ALS, Gib was drinking a glass of Coke at a board meeting when someone cracked a joke. He burst into peals of laughter, inhaled the soda, coughed, and sprayed it over everyone. Afterward he said to Marcia: "I was very embarrassed. I don't know why I did that. It wasn't even a particularly funny joke!"

It is possible that this uncontrollable laughter was the first sign that Gib was developing ALS. Loss of control of emotional reactions is often a symptom of bulbar ALS, since the neurons that control the muscles of the face, mouth, and throat play an important role in the outward expression of emotions. One name given by neurologists to this symptom is *emotional lability*. I prefer to call it *emotional incontinence*, because the involuntary laughter—and more commonly, crying—is rather like urinary incontinence, where the patient has no warning and suddenly wets himself.

Because of the exhaustion, Gib took a six-month leave of absence from Barnett Bank and stayed at home, working on his financial advice column and *Ka Ching*. He returned to the Mayo Clinic in February 2003, where for the first time he was seen by a neurologist. He found that Gib's tongue was shriveled and not moving well, causing him to slur his speech. This was a sign that many of the motor neurons in the bulbar region at the back of the brain had died. In ALS, when a muscle shows the first sign of atrophy, about half of its lower motor neurons are already gone.

The Mayo Clinic neurologists arranged an EMG (electromyogram), where the doctor puts needles into the muscles, looking for electrical signs of damage to the lower motor neurons. They found a hint of damage to the motor neurons supplying Gib's arm muscles. They also did an MRI (magnetic resonance imaging) scan of the brain, looking for signs of a stroke or brain tumor, and found nothing abnormal. They did a lot of blood tests, looking for any vitamin deficiency, hormone imbalance, or toxin that might have caused the symptoms, and again found nothing abnormal.

At the end of the visit, the Mayo doctors told Gib they thought he had ALS. Gib described the process in an interview later published in the *Key West Citizen*, under the headline FULL LIFE AHEAD: ESTATE PLANNER GIB PETERS TALKS ABOUT DYING—AND LIVING—ONE DAY AT A TIME:

"They eliminated every other possibility," said Peters. "Eleven or twelve doctors took a piece of me and tested it. Then, a doctor met me and Marcia. He was the appointed loser, the one who must have drawn the short straw, but he was obviously practiced at it. He said they were 'almost entirely convinced' that it was ALS," recounted Peters, "but my wife, being a nurse, already knew what was going on. Once he said Lou Gehrig's disease, then it registered with me. Is that bad? Is it fatal? What will be the cause of my death?"

The answer was: "The first thing was the dying of the nerves between your brain and your tongue. Then the nerves and muscles in the rest of his body will die. Your heart and brain will be uninvolved, but your body will atrophy. Your diaphragm will no longer work and you'll lose the ability to speak and swallow. There is no cure. It is always fatal."

"They can put tubes in to help me," said Peters. "They can put me on an artificial breathing machine. At some point, I or my family will have to accept the ventilator, or else refuse it and then I'll die. The doctor said that in the end, you or your family will have to decide to pull the plug."

Gib and Marcia flew back from the Mayo Clinic, hardly saying a word as they tried to come to grips with what this diagnosis meant for them and their children. Gib was in shock, but when he reached home he sat down with his children to tell them he had ALS. They all cried together, and everyone was pretty quiet for the next few days, moping around the house with long faces. Marcia was also in shock but had to carry on with her home nursing agency. Looking back, she realized that she never had the time to mourn the diagnosis.

For a month after returning from the Mayo Clinic with his death sentence, Gib was like an automaton. He had always known intellectually that he had to die, but now he was faced with the reality. He did not know exactly when he would die, but it was in a finite and probably short time. He watched TV without really seeing it. He spent a lot of time on the back patio, looking at the canal and mangrove marsh beyond. He spent a lot of time sleeping. Sometimes in the afternoon, while he lay awake in their bedroom studying the palms in the backyard, Marcia would crawl into bed beside him and hold him as they both cried. His four children, all living and working elsewhere in Florida, would get together on the phone for tearful mutual support.

Gib was depressed and shut himself off emotionally from Marcia and his friends. To them he appeared aloof and withdrawn. Most of his friends didn't know how to deal with this, but Bill Schwessinger was not to be denied. He went knocking on Gib's door and insisted on visiting with him. In fact, Gib seemed to welcome the opportunity to open his thoughts to his old friend. They talked on and on for an hour or more about how he was facing death. Bill continued to call on Gib at least once a week, and they would talk about everything under the sun. It was obviously good psychotherapy for Gib.

In June 2003 Gib came to my office at the Kessenich Family MDA ALS Center. My center at the Miller School of Medicine in the University of Miami specializes in the multidisciplinary care of patients with ALS, and in research to find the cause and cure of the disease. *Multidisciplinary* means that we have nurses, physical and occupational therapists, respiratory therapists, swallowing experts, nutritionists, and psychologists, all devoted to the many needs of the ALS patient and his family.

My first impression of Gib was of a man about my age and height, ruggedly handsome and nattily dressed, with short white hair and a ruddy face. Despite the gravity of the situation, he talked with a good deal of humor. I could tell immediately that he was a really nice person.

My heart always sinks when one of my doctors-in-training tells me that the patient she is presenting to me is "a nice man." Neurologists believe that ALS patients are "nicer" than the average patient, and our research has helped to explain this. We interviewed the spouses of fifty ALS patients about the character of their loved one many years before the development of the first symptom of ALS. Then we compared the results with interviews of the spouses of a control group of patients with other diseases, like cancer and multiple sclerosis. Compared to the control group, ALS patients scored higher as "givers" and lower as "complainers" in the years before the development of disease. A patient with ALS often thinks first of the burden that the illness is going to produce for his spouse, rather than the effect of the disease on himself. Perhaps the genes for "niceness" are related to the genes that predispose people to getting ALS.

As Gib described how the condition had come on, I recognized that his speech was slurred. He told me that at times he would choke while drinking. When I examined him, I found that his pronunciation of difficult phrases like "Methodist Episcopal" was slurred as if he were drunk. I saw his wasted tongue. When I tapped on his lips, jaw, arms, and legs with my rubber tendon hammer, I found a much greater movement than is normal. These increased reflexes, as they are called, are an indication of damage to the upper motor neurons running from the brain down to the spinal cord; they drive the lower motor neurons that send "wires" called *axons* to the muscles of the body and limbs.

There was no doubt in my mind that he was in the early stage of bulbar ALS. I told him and his wife, Marcia, my conclusions. Gib said that the Mayo neurologists had told them the same thing and that he and Marcia had come to terms with what this implied: that he had less than two years to live.

Marcia, a petite, svelte, and pretty woman with light-brown shoulder-length hair, had remained in the background as I interviewed Gib. They held hands and clearly loved each other dearly, but she did not talk much. When I later learned that Marcia was a nurse, I was surprised that she did not take a more aggressive role in the consultation.

Much later, when I met her friends, they told me that she was usually very outgoing and the life and soul of the party. When I asked her about this, she admitted that she had been hiding the terrible distress she felt about Gib's ALS; she had looked after a number of patients with ALS and knew the prognosis. She also said that it was Gib's illness, not hers, and that it was for him to decide how he wanted to handle it. She did not want her professional knowledge to interfere with her ability to be his wife.

I believe that it is always important for patients to have hope. Miracles do happen in medicine and doctors are not always right. So I said, "You must not believe everything you read on the Internet. Half of ALS patients live more than three years from their first symptoms. In fact, I have a patient who has a very benign form of the disease, and he is still working after forty years. And then there is the case of Stephen Hawking, who has survived with ALS for more than forty-five years. In addition, I have seen five patients recover from what appeared to all us neurologists to be definite ALS." Like every patient to whom I have given this speech, Gib was astounded. "Why did no one tell me that? What chance do I have of recovering? What was special about those patients who recovered?"

I answered as best I could: "I wish I knew! Though the chance of recovery is extremely slim, in 5 to 10 percent of patients the condition seems to burn itself out. The disease bottoms out and stops progressing." That information seemed to help Gib, though Marcia looked skeptical. I next told them that at present only one drug, Riluzole, is available to treat ALS. The medication slows the progression of the disease by about 20 percent, though it does not do what all of us would want: stop the disease from getting any worse. Riluzole is very expensive, but I told Gib and Marcia that I would take it if I had ALS.

I spoke to Gib about research into the cause and treatment of ALS and suggested that he might like to take part in clinical research trials of new drugs. I think it is very important for patients to take part in clinical trials. They gain the benefit of being the first to receive a possibly effective drug, as well as the hope that the drug may help them and the feeling that through research they are fighting the damned disease. I suggested a new drug that slowed a form of ALS in mice and was now being tested in patients.

Gib and Marcia were enthusiastic about joining the study and signed up for a yearlong trial of this drug, which required him to come to see me every month for testing. Neither he nor any of us on the clinical research team would know whether he was receiving the active drug or a placebo. This is the only way to discover whether a drug works or is harmful. The placebo reaction can be very strong, and patients who think they are getting the active drug may subconsciously do better for a while.

Gib refused to lie down and accept the inevitable prognosis of ALS. He was going to celebrate life, live it to the hilt, and make use of every moment that he had left.

From: Gib Peters
To: All my family and friends
Subject: "And these are my marks"

In February 2003 I complained to Dr. Ellie Gerth about a slight speech slur and a curious emotional instability. I'd sob over Hallmark cards and double over with laughter reading bumper stickers. He ruled out stroke and insanity and sent me up to Rochester Mayo Clinic for a weeklong exam. Thirteen doctors poked and prodded and then drew straws to see who would tell me the bad news. The short straw said, "You've got ALS." Marcia gasped. She knew what amyotrophic lateral sclerosis was. Lou Gehrig's disease. "What in hell is ALS?" I asked. He said, "No known cause, no known cure. You have two or maybe three years. Go home and enjoy life."

For a month or so after Marcia and I returned from the Mayo Clinic, I wallowed in self-pity and cloistered depression until it became obvious even to me that I was mired in a sucking whirlpool of self-destruction. And my family and friends were taking the brunt of it. We were, it seemed, going through the first phases of grieving for the loss that was to come. I decided that nobody was going to lead us out of this but me. I had to brighten up, face the facts, and make the most of what I had left, for my sake and that of my family and friends. "OK, that's enough," I decided. "Got to get a plan together for the rest of my life. Do something."

I've come to grips with my mortality now, and I can tell you, I feel blessed. I have asked my family to let love and life flow like never before. And they certainly have. Birthdays, cruises, long weekends, phone calls by the hundreds, and even the blessed news of new life to come: One of my daughters is pregnant.

Last month, my son, Mike, and son-in-law, George, took me 185 miles down the Colorado River through the Grand Canyon on a raft. It was exciting and humbling. I reached out and brushed past rocks at the river's edge that were formed two billion years ago—one-third the age of Earth itself.

Further up the canyon wall and more recent in time, a granite boulder on a broad ledge revealed a glyph of a stick man carefully chipped into the surface some nine hundred years before. The person who made it stood exactly where I was standing, hearing the river roar as I heard it now, breathing the canyon air as I was breathing it, carefully making his mark for me to see. It said, "I was here. This is who I am." I ran my finger across the grooves and tried to imagine who he was, what he feared, who he loved, and how he died. The answers didn't come, of course, but I felt that I had made human contact fifty generations back in time. I was moved. And I'm a better man for it.

A few days later, much deeper into the canyon where the walls towered a thousand feet overhead, I found impressions in the rocks of sea life that lived a billion years before, a sixth of the life of the Earth itself. A simple sea animal fossil among thousands of others around it, but it was the mark of a living thing past and it had its own simple message: "I was here. This is my mark. You are there because of me." I was awed. How much life and how much death had passed since that time? This very example of ancient life might have been my—our—progenitor. The possibility, however infinitesimal, astounded me.

I was reminded of the unimaginable expanse of time over which our Earth had evolved and the billions of life forms that existed since the life of that fossil. And the inescapable fact that every one, every single life form had died or was about to die. I had been given life, and with it the chance to make the smallest of contributions to those who would follow. Had I done so? What was my "mark"? Would it be seen?

I lay awake that night in my bedroll, looking up through the slot in the earth that was the Grand Canyon. I studied the brilliant swirl of stars that was spinning away from us. Our own Spiral Galaxy, the Milky Way. And what lay beyond our galaxy? Millions more galaxies, we are told. And what's beyond those? God's heaven, perhaps? Or just more space without matter? So much to understand. So little time to understand it. I rolled over in my bedroll and wiggled my hip into the sand for a more comfortable position. But sleep wouldn't come. My mind reeled with questions, and I dug deep for the few answers I had once learned but had long forgotten.

One question kept coming back: Where did it all come from? All the stars, moons, gas, and unseen matter all around us? This is what I remembered: Einstein told us that matter can be converted to energy and energy back to matter; but neither can be destroyed. Then Stephen Hawking said that every atom of the universe was created within a nanosecond of the Big Bang some twelve billion years ago—from a single small point of matter, far smaller than a single atom. Where did that speck come from? Well, I must have missed that lecture; I don't remember or wasn't told.

I rolled over onto the other hip, wiggled into the sand again, and tried once more for sleep. OK, how did that single speck of matter explode into all the rocks and gas that make up the universe today? My notes are vague on that too, but I recall the cosmologists saying that it was exploded with a "charge" of nearly infinite, pure energy. Well, where did all that energy come from? God, perhaps?

Oh, how I yearn to believe it was God's energy. That he said, "OK, it's time to start the universe. I'll zap the speck with a little energy, convert the energy into atoms of star dust that will hurtle outward into space forever, spinning off into galaxies of solar systems that will eventually support life. Odds are, intelligent life will sprout and try to deal with its meaning and with my existence. That's when the game will become really interesting." I call this Gib's Catechism. After flying around in the form of rocks, gas, or water for twelve billion years, a few of the atoms that were created at that first moment became . . . me. I lay and wondered that night, just as he expected: "What does it mean? Is there a God? Do I exist as a direct result of His design and from His pure energy?" I hoped so. I believed so. I slept.

Now I'm home. And I ask myself, "Where's MY mark? What will I leave behind that will help make someone after me a better person?" My contributions to the world have been neither profound nor heroic. They are but a few drops in an ocean of thoughts and deeds left behind by untold millions who came before me. I think of these things now. And I'm coming to understand that my true marks, the things that I helped create to make the world a better place, are my children. Beautiful like their mother, strong like me, and with passion and fire from somewhere in our French-Canadian and Irish ancestry. Through them, and through their children's children after them, I leave my mark. These are who I am.

Gib

I n October 2003 Gib began talking of taking *Ka Ching* on a circumnavigation of the eastern United States. Thinking about a long sea trip was his way of dealing with the diagnosis of ALS. His route would take him from Key West up the Atlantic Intracoastal Waterway (ICW), along the east coasts of Florida, Georgia, South and North Carolina, Virginia, and Maryland. Then he would head north up Chesapeake Bay, through the Chesapeake & Delaware Canal, and down Delaware Bay to Cape May at the southern tip of New Jersey. From there he would pick up the ICW to Manasquan Inlet, New Jersey, after which he faced a thirty-mile stretch of open Atlantic Ocean leading to New York harbor.

From New York he planned to go up the Hudson River, through the Erie Canal and Great Lakes, down the salubriously named Chicago Sanitary and Ship Canal to the Mississippi, and from there to the Gulf of Mexico and the Gulf ICW, to finish his odyssey back at Key West. This was a short version of the "full circumnavigation," known to cruising sailors as the Great Loop. The complete journey of 7,500 nautical miles adds the segment from New York up the east coasts of Connecticut, Rhode Island, Massachusetts, New Hampshire, Maine, and Nova Scotia, round the Gaspé Peninsula of Quebec, and then up the Saint Lawrence River to the Great Lakes.

To avoid summer hurricanes along the southeast coast and winter ice in the north, Great Loopers start from Florida in the early spring and spend the summer traversing the Great Lakes. With fall approaching, they head south down the Illinois and Mississippi Rivers, and arrive back in Key West around November. This was what Gib had in mind for his odyssey of self-discovery.

The history of the Intracoastal, affectionately known as The Ditch, goes back to the earliest European explorers of North America, who discovered the series of navigable channels, tidal streams, bays, and sounds that ran along much of the Eastern Seaboard, protected from the hazards of the Atlantic Ocean by a series of natural barrier islands.

The Florida Keys, the southernmost part of this chain, were formed from coral reefs near the edge of the Florida Platform. The Florida Peninsula as we know it from today's maps is only that part of the Florida Platform that lies above the current sea level. The whole platform is much broader, 350 miles wide and 450 miles long. It extends a hundred miles westward into the Gulf of Mexico and ten miles south of the Florida Keys toward Cuba. The Florida Platform rises up from the surrounding 10,000-foot-deep abyss. To the west lie the depths of the Gulf of Mexico, and to the east those of the Atlantic Ocean. Coral reefs that formed the Florida Keys, and other reefs now lying to the south and east of the Keys, grew as the sea level rose and fell over the eons.

The origin of the other barrier islands is less clear. One theory is that sand and silt from the center of the continent were washed down the east-flowing rivers into the Atlantic and then carried southward by prevailing currents to create the series of north-south oriented barrier islands. Another theory is that wave action pushed sand from the Atlantic continental shelf toward the mainland, building up the series of islands. A third theory is that the low-lying marshland near the coast was flooded as the sea level rose at the end of the last Ice Age, cutting off the mainland from the higher coastal ridges, which became a string of barrier islands.

Whatever their origin, these barrier islands provided early settlers with a protected passage up and down the East Coast. But it was not continuous, nor was it deep enough for large boats. The first Congress of the new United States of America, recognizing the importance of navigation to the country, passed a number of acts to improve the harbors, navigable rivers, and waterways. Federal enabling acts provided money for Georgia to improve Savannah Harbor, for Maryland to improve Baltimore Harbor, and for Pennsylvania to build harbors on the Delaware River. Commercial companies were formed to supplement the efforts of the government and to connect various parts of the Inland Passage, though the history of these ventures was one of grand ideas and financial failures.

The U.S. Army Corps of Engineers was established in 1802, and soon thereafter Congress authorized the construction of coastal fortifications, lighthouses, harbors, and navigation channels. In 1808 Albert Gallatin, the U.S. Treasury Secretary, drew up a comprehensive plan to provide the young nation with an essential infrastructure of roads and canals. He proposed the construction of an inland waterway from Boston to Georgia that he thought would take only ten years to complete. In fact, construction of the ICW went on piecemeal for over 150 years, and even today portions of Gallatin's dream remain unfinished.

By 1830 two important connectors were completed. The Dismal Swamp Canal connected Chesapeake Bay and Albemarle Sound, and the Chesapeake and Delaware Canal linked the northern ends of Chesapeake and Delaware Bays. The C&D

Canal alone cut more than three hundred miles off the sea route from Philadelphia to Baltimore and soon became a major route for commercial shipping. The C&D Canal has been expanded several times since then and is now 450 feet wide and thirty-five feet deep, large enough for oceangoing vessels and barges. From 1850 the Army Corps of Engineers and private companies dredged channels and built canals to create the Atlantic ICW. Linking major bodies of water like Biscayne Bay in Florida, the Pamlico and Albemarle Sounds in North Carolina, and the Delaware and Chesapeake Bays, the Atlantic Intracoastal is an almost complete inland waterway from Key West to Maine.

Nowadays the Atlantic ICW is very different from the original channel that ran through virgin territory, connecting the major cities of Boston, New York, Philadelphia, Richmond, and Savannah. It now runs by the "flesh pots" of Miami Beach and the Jersey shore. In its early years, sailors on the ICW were entranced by open vistas full of wildlife. Now there are far fewer birds, and their songs are often replaced by the noise of industrial plants, marinas, and trucks crossing the bridges spanning the waterway. Real estate along the waterway has become very expensive. Mega-million-dollar homes, high-rise condominiums, and luxury hotels line some of the route, and luxury boats fill the docks and marinas, though there are still spots along the waterway that remain serene and relatively unchanged.

The ICW is tidal, with many inlets to the Atlantic Ocean. The salt or brackish water is generally clear, except where big ships stir up the mud with propellers that are only a few feet above the dredged bottom. The Army Corps of Engineers is charged with maintaining a channel with a minimum depth of twelve feet and a minimum width of one hundred feet, but in many places the channel can be as shallow as five feet and as narrow as fifty feet.

Gib would be navigating the ICW aboard *Ka Ching*, a stubby twenty-nine-foot Wellcraft Sportsbridge built around 1980. She had a three-foot bow pulpit that held the windlass and a swim platform aft that carried the inflatable dinghy and several storage bins. Her beam was ten feet and her draft four feet. She had a glass-enclosed cabin with a control flybridge above. When Gib was sitting on the bridge shaded by the bimini, he was about eleven feet above the waterline. Forward glass panes and lateral and rear roll-down transparent vinyl panels could enclose the flybridge in bad weather. A six-foot vertical bridge ladder led from the flybridge to the main deck. Gib had to climb and descend this ladder many times a day.

The stern of the boat was an open deck, also covered by a collapsible bimini, where there was a small round breakfast table and a couple of wicker armchairs. Two Chevy V8 350-cubic-inch inboard marine diesel engines and a generator for power for the air conditioner and other electrical equipment on the boat were housed beneath the stern deck and accessed through lift-up hatches.

The main cabin, on the same level as the rear deck, was entered through a door with a glass window. The cabin was nine feet long. Aft on the starboard side was the communication center and a three-by-three-foot chart table, with benches fore and aft. Gib used the chart table for the radio and his laptop computer. Forward of the chart table bench was a work surface with stowage beneath. Aft on the port side, immediately inside the entrance door, was the enclosed head and shower. Forward of this was the galley, consisting of a sink, a small refrigerator below, the range, and a work surface with cupboards below. The cabin had windows all round. Forward and amidships, between the two work surfaces and the forward window, was the entrance to the small sleeping area, with a pair of bunks tucked into the vee of the bow. *Ka Ching* was nothing if not snug, but Gib had all the space he needed.

Gib had been slowly fixing up the boat since he bought her in 2000. When he decided to take *Ka Ching* on a trip through the ICW, he realized that he needed this refit to be completed before he started his odyssey. He had already replaced the old diesel engines with a pair of factory-reconditioned engines, but all manner of other things still needed repair. He rewired the whole boat. He built an automatic steering gear that would keep the boat on a compass course so that he would not have to keep his hands on the steering wheel all the time. He called this Iron Mike.

The total cost of fixing up *Ka Ching* and of the voyage on the ICW was well in excess of $100,000, and this expenditure ate up much of Marcia and Gib's financial reserves. She was very supportive, but when a large box arrived shortly before Gib was due to depart, she asked what it was. When Gib replied that he had bought a plasma screen TV for the boat, she blew her stack. The box went back the next day, unopened.

When Gib shared with Bill Schwessinger his idea of making the Great Loop trip, Bill said, "You'll have to take someone with you. It would be too much for you alone. It's a physically taxing journey even for the able-bodied! It'll take you eight or nine months to complete, so you'll go though some pretty cold weather up around New York and Chicago."

"No way!" said Gib. "I'm going to do the trip single-handed. I want time to think about life and to enjoy what I have left."

Bill could not control himself. "You must be out of your mind! I don't think you could even get to New York on your own." Gib was not deterred by Bill's outburst. Later he declined many offers from friends to join him on the trip. His explanation was that he wanted to have time to himself to think. He did ask Marcia to go with him, but she needed to keep her home nursing agency running to pay the expenses.

In March 2004, when Gib told me about his plan to do the Great Loop, I reviewed in my mind's eye the tempo of progression that his ALS had taken over the last nine months and projected what was likely to happen in the next nine months.

In June 2003 he had only a little slurring of his speech and occasional choking. By November 2003 Gib was drooling like a baby. As the ALS caused more bulbar motor neurons to die, the weakening muscles in his tongue and throat made it progressively more difficult for him to swallow. Gib was also losing weight, and poor nutrition causes ALS to accelerate. In January 2004 I arranged for a PEG tube to be put into his stomach to bypass his mouth and throat. Gib was briefly anesthetized, and a 3/4-inch-diameter plastic tube was inserted through his belly into his stomach. It is not a painful procedure, and I always tell patients that they'll still be able to do most things as usual: bathe, go to social events, have sex!

By March 2004 Gib's speech had become so bad that I recommended a speech synthesizer, an apparatus that converts typed words into synthetic speech. His right arm was also beginning to weaken. Projecting forward, I thought that in six months his arms would be useless and he would be having difficulty breathing. I feared that in nine months, without a ventilator, Gib might be dead.

I did not share this dire prediction with Gib in so many words, but I did say, "Gib, you have to be mad! The idea of you taking a single-handed boat trip to New York is crazy. It would be difficult enough for you to make this trip with someone else helping. You certainly could not do it alone."

I then said something that Gib would hold over me in the coming months: "I think you must be developing a deterioration of the frontal parts of your brain that we call frontotemporal dementia. This is often associated with bulbar ALS and tends to impair the patient's judgment." Gib was not to be deterred. With a twinkle in his eye, he mumbled, "Doc, I'm going to do it!"

As usual, Marcia had kept in the background during this conversation, but I asked what she thought of the plan. "Gib can be very obstinate when he gets something into his head," was her only response. So I said to Gib, "Look! It's your life. Obviously, I can't stop you from going. But you are enrolled in our research drug trial, and you must come back to see me every month if you want to continue. That will give us both an opportunity to see how the ALS is progressing. If you become so weak that in my judgment you are a danger to yourself and others, I will tell you and Marcia." And that was how we left it.

Marcia understood only too well the nature of ALS and its likely course, both from patients she had looked after and from research on the Internet. She began to look for alternative medicine treatments, as do many relatives of patients with ALS. Gib, on the other hand, adopted a more fatalistic attitude and was not interested in Marcia's suggestions about new treatments for him to try. His response was always, "Whatever." Marcia read that someone had said magnets might help, and got little pocket magnets for all Gib's clothes. She even fit a machine under the bed that rotated a magnet all night long. He said, "I don't know if it works, but when I get up in the morning my dick points north!"

~~~~~

Gib intended to leave for his voyage up the ICW in March 2004, but it took forever to get *Ka Ching* ready. His progressing weakness added to the delay. When I saw him in April 2004 for the research trial, his speech had deteriorated and he often had to write to make himself understood. His neck muscles had weakened further, and whenever he leaned forward his head would drop onto his chest. I gave him a prescription for a soft sorbo-rubber collar, but like most patients he found this uncomfortable and preferred to hold up his head with one hand under his chin as though deep in thought.

Because Gib was drooling all the time, he held a tissue or a towel to his lips. He asked if I could help reduce the dribbling. I tried all the medications that dry up saliva, but none worked very well for him. In a frustrated and unguarded moment, I told him that drooling was only a social inconvenience. When he returned home to his computer, he took me to task for this in no uncertain terms.

From: Gib Peters
To: Dr. Walter Bradley
Subject: Drooling

Psychologically, I'm retreating from social contact because of the embarrassment about the drooling and the reaction of my friends is quite damaging. I have begged off meeting old friends or having them see me because of it, and, as I think about it, drooling may have contributed to my decision to be alone on *Ka Ching*, away from friends and family. The reaction of those who see me struggle with it when I try to speak or simply sit quietly and "drip and wipe" is quite obvious. They don't understand it and know it embarrasses me. So they absent themselves for the company of others.

Of less importance, but nevertheless a factor, is that when I'm working with papers, food preparation, keyboard, workshop projects, etc., the flow of saliva on my work-product is, to say the least, disconcerting. I find myself avoiding such projects because of the risk of fouling my work.

This is not a plea for more drastic measures, but rather a suggestion that the problem can and for me does have more serious consequences than what you may suspect or that others may have told you. I hope my comments help.

Warmest regards.
Gib

In late April 2004, Gib took *Ka Ching* on a trial run to the Marquesas Keys, thirty miles west of Key West. Marcia went with him, but Gib had not expected her to sit back and do nothing. He was pretty unhappy about the lack of help, but Marcia wanted to see if he really *could* manage the boat alone.

Gib realized he would be unable to talk to people while under way, so he set up an Internet connection on his laptop computer using his cell phone. This would allow him to be in constant e-mail contact with his family. Through this link he would be able to book a slip in a marina, order service and parts for the boat, and book cars and airline tickets for journeys to Miami to see me for the drug trial.

Gib's laptop computer became his connection to the outside world. He inundated friends and family with over two thousand e-mail messages in the next seven months. Initially his communications were just with Marcia and his children, his close friends, and me and my staff. But Gib was a born writer and humorist, and soon his friends and family began to ask if they could forward these e-mails to other friends. Some of these new contacts wrote to congratulate him, offering heartfelt best wishes for his odyssey. Several responses came from other ALS patients. By the end of the trip, more than a hundred people were on his e-mail list server.

Eventually, all the essential preparations aboard *Ka Ching* were complete. Gib was, at last, ready to set out on his great adventure. Gib and Marcia organized a send-off party a few days before the actual departure. All of their friends attended, offering items that he might find useful on the voyage, like books to read and life vests. Although there was a lot of backslapping, everyone worried about his safety on the odyssey.

Despite Gib's insistence on taking the trip alone, Marcia suggested he bring a cat for some companionship. They realized that a grown cat would not adapt to the boat, but a kitten would grow up on the boat and acclimatize quickly. At the NSPCA Gib was like a kid in a candy store; first he wanted this one, then he wanted that one. After a considerable time, he picked what Marcia thought were the two ugliest kittens in the whole shelter and took them home.

Several of Gib's friends said to Marcia: "How can you let him go? It's going to be dangerous, and he shouldn't be going off alone." Others thought that Gib was selfish to stay away from Marcia and the children for so long. "I am very upset that he is taking himself away from me for seven months when I have so little time left with him," Kim said to her mother. Lisa said, "I just know he's going to do it. He's stubborn, just like me!"

The family was supportive, but they insisted that Gib send them an e-mail every night, giving them his position and an update on how he was doing.

To ease their minds, he explained to friends and family all that went into making *Ka Ching* seaworthy.

From: Gib Peters
To: All my family and friends
Subject: The making of *Ka Ching*

Ka Ching is a sturdy vessel made by Wellcraft. Twenty-nine feet in length, if you don't count the bowsprit holding the ground tackle or the dive platform now crowded with a tilt-up inflatable dinghy and large plastic storage containers. Her beam is ten feet, and her draft to the propeller tips is four feet, fully loaded. I've set the shallow depth alarm at seven feet, which has saved my butt on several occasions cruising up the ICW.

I worked full-time for most of a year getting her ready for my voyage, beginning shortly after I was diagnosed with ALS in February 2003. To get over my depression, I decided that I wanted to take a long voyage in *Ka Ching*.

God, I'd love to single-hand a forty-foot sailboat to Cuba, South America, or even around the Horn, as my friend Nance Frank did some years ago. Well, she didn't quite take on the Horn, but she did navigate the Straits of Magellan just north of the Cape, single-handed, from west to east—no small feat for any sailor. What a woman!

But it was a tired old motor vessel that I owned, in much need of repair. I used it once every six months to ferry my gang of ten out to the Key West reefs for lobster or diving, and then only if I could get her started. How could I take THAT heap of junk to Cuba? Sailboats don't have fuel problems, while *Ka Ching* sucks it up like a flushing toilet, at a gallon a mile. But it was too late to consider trading her in for a sailing vessel, and besides, I was simply not strong enough any longer to haul sheets and halyards single-handed. "How about a trip with fuel within reach the whole way?" The ICW was the obvious answer, and the more I thought about the idea, the less depressed I became. "Maybe all the way up to the St. Lawrence, take a left turn into the Great Lakes, and back south down the Mississippi to home?"

Well, anything past Florida is sheer speculation. I can claim a small victory even if everything falls apart after that. The St. Lawrence is a long way away and quite desolate; the Great Lakes can become rougher than the Atlantic Ocean in a severe storm; and the Mississippi River is spotted with submerged hazards that would curl up my twin blades like potato chips. So where am I going? North, that's where. Lewis and Clark went west to find a water route to the Pacific, knowing little about the country they would cover. I'm going north, knowing little about my route and my destination, to find . . . me!

Ka Ching had to be made seaworthy for whatever lay ahead, and made as comfortable as such a vessel would allow. Luckily, by the time of my diagnosis, I had already man-handled two replacement Chevy V8 engines into her and replaced two one-hundred-gallon gas tanks under her afterdeck. I was stronger then; I couldn't do it now. But literally hundreds of systems and gadgets still didn't work. So every day, eight or ten hours a day for almost a year, I worked with purpose and joy. The therapy was wonderful for both body and mind and for the morale of my family. As I pulled old wire through the bilge, replaced rusted steering pinions, and sanded and painted old gel coat, I'd try to imagine the challenges and needs for such a trip, and to find the answer to a re-emerging question: "Why in the hell am I doing this?" For now, it was good enough to say, "Because I can."

My departure, initially set for March 1, 2004, was delayed twice because *Ka Ching* simply wasn't ready. March was selected at the suggestion of my good friend Bill Schwessinger, who cautioned me about the summer heat in Florida and the cold in the North. But by May it became obvious that the ALS was moving faster than it had during the first year after my diagnosis, and that any thought of delaying until next year just wasn't in the cards. My neck and shoulder muscles were becoming weaker, and I was all but speechless, which worried me about how I would communicate with other vessels, the bridge tenders, and the Coast Guard if necessary. It was time to go. Even though I still had three pages of to-dos to make *Ka Ching* reasonably safe and comfortable, I'd take my tool shop along on the trip and devote a few hours a day to whittling away the list.

And so on May 19, 2004, with Marcia, my friend Bill Schwessinger, and Calvin on the seawall, I pushed off for a voyage of self-discovery with a small prayer: "Please God, be patient just a little bit longer."

Love to all.
Gib

G ib finally set off from the dock at his house on Riviera Channel on Wednesday, May 19, 2004. Marcia called Bill Schwessinger to say that Gib was about to leave, and Bill dropped everything and rushed over. He wanted to cast off the lines and wish Gib Godspeed, even though he still feared that he would not survive the trip—that he would fall and injure himself or else tumble into the water and drown. Marcia secretly thought that Gib would be back in two weeks.

Gib Peters, on the other hand, was on the voyage of a lifetime, a voyage that he had dreamed about from the time he was diagnosed with ALS. He had no doubt about his abilities and fully expected to complete his circumnavigation of the eastern United States. As he steered the brave little boat *Ka Ching* eastward up the Riviera Canal, Gib was excited about the adventures that lay ahead. Seated on the captain's bench on the flybridge, he surveyed his vessel. The Stars and Stripes flew proudly from an aft stanchion on the starboard side, and the blue flag of the Conch Republic from a forward one on the port side. The inflatable dinghy was hiked up on the swim platform astern, together with a couple of storage chests. He was king of all he surveyed.

Gib turned *Ka Ching* south into Cow Key Canal and headed for the open sea. The route he had selected for the first part of the journey was northeast up Hawk Channel, which Keys dwellers call the "outside" or "oceanside" route. It runs between the Keys and the offshore reefs and follows a gentle curve as it turns toward Miami, 150 miles to the north. The offshore reefs protect this channel from the worst of the Atlantic swells.

The first few days of the trip provided a shakedown for the boat and also for its captain. Gib was not confident that his new Chevy V8 diesels were up to the task of traveling five thousand miles or more and was afraid to challenge them too soon. He set the throttles at 1,500 rpm for a speed of seven knots. He worked the helm and controls for the twin engines with his hands, but they soon became tired, particularly the right one. He rested his knees against the wheel and found he could not only hold the boat steady but also steer it.

Setting a course of 078 degrees, he passed Boca Chica Naval Station three miles to port, then Cudjoe Key, Sugarloaf, and the Lower Keys. The Florida Keys are a hundred-mile-long chain of islands strung like pearls along the Overseas Highway. This is the beginning of US 1, which runs all the way to Fort Kent in Maine.

Gib was an experienced boater, but this was the first long trip that he had taken, the first single-handed trip of this magnitude, and the first trip when he had to anticipate progressive loss of strength due to ALS. He approached the odyssey as a challenge— not so much to himself, but rather as a challenge by Gib Peters to the disease. I do not think that he had much thought about the perils that might befall him, nor the frustrations that he would experience. This was his final battle, his final goal, and he was going to do it, come hell or high water!

Soon he left the built-up islands around Key West and passed the much less developed Lower Keys. Near Channel Key, in the

Middle Keys, he switched to the "inside" or "gulfside" route that hugs the Florida Bay side of the Keys. The inside route is more protected, but in many places it is less than six feet deep, posing the risk of grounding. The inside route provides the boater with some of Florida's most beautiful vistas: many undeveloped islands, ringed by mangroves and topped by low scrubby trees, with only a few resorts and marinas dotted along the way.

After a few days, *Ka Ching* was in the Upper Keys, cruising beside the touristy islands of Islamorada and Key Largo, where it is now difficult to find the tiki bars and open vistas that used to be the attraction of these lovely islands.

For the first ten days of his odyssey, Gib could not work the e-mail link from his computer through his cell phone. Marcia knew that he was all right because he used the cell phone to call her every evening, though she found it very difficult to understand him. For the rest of us, we did not know if the silence meant that he had suffered an accident and drowned. We were greatly relieved when Gib finally fixed the problem and sent the first e-mail of his journey.

From: Gib Peters
To: All my family and friends
Subject: At last

At last I have the e-mail going. I am anchored this morning eight hundred feet northwest of Pumpkin Key, off Key Largo. The trip has been a breeze so far; no major problems, although I've been kept busy with minor electrical and mechanical glitches that popped up along the way. My routine is beginning to take shape . . . by the time I get to New York, it should be firmed up.

If you haven't heard, Marcia was able to find a live cat for me . . . in fact two; they are six weeks old, potty trained, and eat continuously. Only one problem: They haven't got names yet. Everything else on the boat has a name, so I guess it's time that the two fuzzy-chinned terrorists I've taken on board have names too. Marcia and I picked them up at the cat pound the week before I left, when they were just six weeks old. I can't swear to the exact age, but I'm captain and I'm declaring their birthdays to be April 10, 2004. They were in a pound cage together and obviously in love with me at first sight (or hungry). I picked them out from the others because their color reminded me of some phenomenally delicious double-chocolate cupcakes my mother used to make for me—glossy black and caramel-brown.

"So, what are they?" I asked the pound lady. "Don't know; let's cop a feel." I was a bit taken aback by her unexpected method of determining the sex of my new kittens, but soon understood that just "looking" wasn't going to yield the information that I required. With the nonchalance of a practiced professional, the pound lady scooped up the nearest kitten, unceremoniously flipped it over. While studying the far wall for inspiration, she gently prodded the squirming bottom. "Hmm, let's see the other one." She repeated the procedure, this time with a frown. "I think . . . yeah, I think that one is a boy and this one is a girl. So you better have them spayed and neutered in six months."

We put our two new treasures into a box with holes and headed for home, but not before stopping for cat food, litter, and collars: one pink, one blue. I took the cat box and the bags of cat stuff directly to the boat. They scrambled out of their cardboard cage and together tentatively explored the afterdeck while I looked for the collars. I picked up the pink one and suddenly realized that I didn't have a clue which kitten was which. And I wasn't about to emulate the cat-lady. They are as close to twins

36

as could be—same marking, colors, size, and manners. So I just put the pink collar on one and the blue on the other. We'll see if it turns out right.

The correct colors can wait, but not their names. So please offer up some imaginative, Key-sie names for my two companions. Winner gets free beer tomorrow.

Love to all.
Gib

~~~~~

From: Walter Bradley
To: Gib Peters
Subject: At last

Good luck on the travels. You are a braver man than I am, Gunga Din! I suggest Faith and Hope for the names of the kittens.

Best wishes.
Wally

As I sent the two names to him, I was thinking about the third of the three martyred virgins, Faith, Hope, and Charity. More than just faith and hope, Gib was going to need a good deal of charity from people along the way if he was to reach his goal. I know that he understood my not-so-subtle message.

~~~~~

North of Key Largo, the Intracoastal Waterway (ICW) passes under US 1 at Jewfish Creek. The old bascule drawbridge had a clearance of only eleven feet when closed, and Gib gesticulated to the bridge keeper to open the bridge to let *Ka Ching* pass.

Jewfish Creek Bridge, now replaced by a new flyover bridge with a sixty-five-foot clearance, is the southernmost of over two hundred bridges of all types that cross the Atlantic ICW. Many are high-clearance bridges that offer no problem for the sailors of small boats, but many others are cantilever bascule bridges, where one or two sections swing upward. Others are swing bridges that rotate on the horizontal plane to allow boats to pass through. All of these "active" bridges are operated by bridge masters. Regular opening times are posted on websites and charts, but at other times the boat captain has to call the bridge master on VHF radio channel 9 or 16. For Gib, who already had difficulty making himself understood, this was an ever-increasing problem.

From Jewfish Creek Bridge, Gib followed the dredged ICW channel across Biscayne Bay to Miami. Passing Brickell and downtown Miami, the view of the condominiums and office buildings reaching fifty stories into the sky is like a miniature Manhattan. Next come the glitzy hotels and condominiums of Miami Beach, Hollywood, and Fort Lauderdale, where the Intracoastal is lined by mega-yachts and houses of the rich and famous.

Some parts of the Intracoastal are very photogenic, and Gib was busy with his camera as he passed northward after the South Florida conurbations. This area is famous for its limpid light, which some say vies with that of Venice. The particular quality of the light seems to come from the sun shining through subtropical humidity and makes the region a mecca for fashion photographers.

From: Gib Peters
To: All my family and friends
Subject: Decision Day

It's 8 a.m. and it must be Wednesday; my meds box has pills in the Wednesday morning spot. I am anchored a half a mile off the ICW in West Palm Beach. My GPS showed no anchor drag last night, and the horizon looks the same as last evening.

And it's decision day. The naming of my completely useless crew, cat 1 and cat 2. Each has slightly different black and brown patterns. I considered it important to determine their gender, so under squeaky, squirmy protest, I turned them both upside down on my lap and attempted a scientific analysis of their behinds, side by side. The one with lighter brown stripes has a bulge that the darker-patterned one does not. Hmm, but which is which? I have to conclude that I can't tell . . . yet. Nevertheless, after considerable thought I've made a decision. Dick Moody suggested Port and Starboard. Others contributed equally appropriate monikers: Mutt and Jeff, Marge and Rita (margarita), and Flotsam and Jetsam. Not wanting to piss off my doctor, I've taken his suggestion of Faith and Hope. The names border on the superstitious, but what the hell, he's probably trying to tell me something. So, dark and stripe-less is Faith, and light-brown stripes is Hope.

Weather looks good as I check the windward horizon, but the weather guessers on channel 3 are making a fuss about very hot temperatures and building thunder-boomers this afternoon. I will get an early start and plan to anchor in one of the many lake areas northward around 2 or 3 p.m. Nevertheless, I'm prepared to drop the windowed bimini sides on the bridge and anchor if things get wild.

The coffee is taking hold, Faith and Hope are brimming with energy and impatience, so I'll get *Ka Ching* fired up and under way up the ICW.

Love to all.
Gib

So the two little terrorists were named Faith and Hope. The kittens became the source of several wonderful stories that Gib sent to his friends while on the trip. I never did get the free beer!

~~~~~

As soon as he was able to e-mail, Gib gave me feedback on his condition. He reminded me that I had told him he was mad to contemplate such an arduous trip and had suggested that perhaps this was a symptom of brain degeneration.

From: Gib Peters
To: Dr. Walter Bradley
Subject: Medical report

Dr. Bradley, greetings from the motor vessel *Ka Ching*. I've traveled up the Keys coast (mostly inside) to the ICW. I'm presently at a marina in Delray Beach. My general health is good and my mood "buoyant." You will recognize how nautical I've become in these few days. The PEG tube is working fine, and I'm on nine to ten cans of Jevity per day to keep my weight from dropping. I have been burning more calories than expected. I seem to have stabilized around 185 pounds. My appetite is good, but I've found that eating virtually anything makes me choke continuously . . . other than rum and coke—funny how smooth that goes down. My speech continues to degrade; now almost unintelligible. I've had to use the radio only once during my trip so far, and the bridge tender I spoke to quickly guessed what I wanted: Raise the damn bridge!

My right arm continues to weaken, although the fingers are still good. My neck muscles are weakening, though if I avoid working all day with my head down, they serve well enough without the soft brace. My left arm is still a 5 out of 5, but I'm noticing some weakening, about where my right arm was a year ago. Breathing is fine. I've taken two memorable falls during the past six months and have become very conscious of each step I take aboard *Ka Ching.*

You'll be glad to know that, in my judgment, my judgment is fine! And I've never lied, either!

Warmest regards.
Gib

~~~~~

From: Gib Peters
To: All my family and friends
Subject: Running aground

Well, it happened: I ran aground in the ICW near Jupiter. One of those storms the weather guesser guessed began building in the northwest, and as the winds freshened I thought I'd be smart and find shelter to drop anchor. Ahead appeared a widening of the channel, surrounded by a string of those ten-million-dollar homes with a few gazebos occupied by old men and twenty-million-dollar women. There was a marina tucked into one corner. So as the temperature dropped, I made a left toward the outermost finger where a half dozen thirty-five-footers were tied up. "Ping, ping, ping." My sonar said to me: "You are at four and a half feet, dimwit! STOP!" But not in time. I felt the blades slash through mud and sand. "Soft aground," I was thirty yards from the channel and fifty yards from those old men and expensive women who were now shifting in their deck chairs for a better view. And yes, the storm was approaching now, with a black ugly bottom dropping lightning bolts to the ground about five miles away.

Being the resourceful, reasoning person that I am, I panicked! How do I get off this mud before the wind pushes me into one of those boats, the shoreline, or, God forbid, rocks. I dropped my bow anchor, broke out the storm anchor, and heaved it over the transom. I jumped into the four feet of water and mud. I carried the bow anchor twenty yards ahead into five to six feet of water, and the stern anchor back another thirty yards. I took a strain on each line and did the most heroic thing I could think of. I called Tow Boat U.S.!

As the little fire-engine-red towboat pulled alongside, the storm evaporated and the wind calmed. And the tide began to rise. "Yeah, pull me off anyway. I can't afford a couple of bent props," I said to the kid. And he did. The tow took one and a half minutes, paperwork took ten minutes, and the bill was $300. But I was on my way again, up the ICW bound for Port St. Lucie, from where I am writing tonight.

Warmest regards to all from Faith and Hope and me.
Gib

Doing laundry on *Ka Ching* was another problem.

From: Gib Peters
To: All my family and friends
Subject: Laundry day

On the first days out of Key West, I rolled my soiled clothing into tight, space-saving lumps and stuffed them into an eight-gallon plastic bag. After a while the bag showed signs of splitting, so I moved it from the forward vee-bunk to the vanity-top in the head and added a second bag. Fourth day out that too began to over-flow with wet jackets, towels, and other stuff that I never thought would have to be washed for the entire trip. A couple of days ago, I decided to forget the whole bag idea. I simply opened the head door and tossed my shorts on a growing pile on the floor. Yesterday I moved everything out to the aft deck and now simply open the cabin door, toss my underwear out, and quickly shut the door for fear of things rolling back into the cabin.

I can hear you now: "How about washing a few things?" Well, I did. Yesterday. Got out my bucket on the aft deck, sloshed up some soapy water, and plunged in an experimental T-shirt. While rubbing and dipping and pissing and moaning, I remembered my mother doing the same thing with my dad's factory work-shirts in the kitchen sink with the luxury of a corrugated washboard. What an innovation that must have been. There is no way these damned drool spots will come out without a washboard.

So I fired the T-shirt back into the pile, looked over the horizon, and wondered where I could find a Laundromat. This morning I identified one at a nearby marina and will launch the dinghy for an important run ashore.

Love to all.
Gib

~~~~~

From: Gib Peters
To: All my family and friends
Subject: PEG tube

I'm anchored just a half-mile from Melbourne, and it's a glorious morning. According to my meds box, it's Saturday. Yesterday's cruise north from Vero was uneventful, except for a fierce summer storm out of the northwest. The boat was pulled off the "road," well anchored and tugging wildly at its reins. Inside, with the A/C, lights, stereo, and a Rum *Ka Ching*, I was satisfied with my victory in this small fight with the elements and content to be living my dream.

So what's a Rum *Ka Ching*?

A little background first. My Lou Gehrig's disease is in its second year after diagnosis in February of 2003. From the slight slurring I noticed six months before that, the disease has progressed to nearly complete paralysis of the tongue and inability to swallow. I see it as a challenge to cheat my ALS by inventing "workarounds" and innovations. Small victories in a war that won't be won.

Victory this time came when Doc Bradley had a PEG tube placed just below the sternum into my stomach for intake of liquid nourishment. Having balanced the joy of tasting and savoring food against the choking, I've resigned myself to liquid tube feedings from now on, without the joy of tasting good food again.

My formula comes in eight-ounce cans and pours like heavy chocolate milk. I've got about 240 cans on board, and I imagine them as being cans of Miller Lite, a slice of pizza, an inch-thick New York strip (medium), and so on. But my evening tot of rum is damn well for real: an eight-ounce can of formula mixed with a double finger of good rum drained right down the old PEG tube. This is a Rum *Ka Ching*. Now that's a bar trick you've got to see!

So, as I was saying, it's a beautiful morning and my two boat kittens, Faith and Hope, are bounding around the afterdeck, trying to pin down a bug of some kind. They are nine weeks old, and I still don't know whether they are sisters or brothers. I'll reserve judgment until they stop chasing bugs and start chasing one another. Ah, the challenges of a captain's duty weigh heavily.

Love to all.
Gib

Gib's PEG tube added another dimension of complexity to the cruise for Gib and Marcia. Every week Marcia had to send a supply of cases of Jevity Plus or Ensure to the harbormaster at the next marina that Gib would be visiting. Without these "care packages," Gib would have starved to death! Since he needed nine or more cans a day, Marcia had to manage the logistics of sending more than three hundred eight-packs of liquid food over the seven months of the journey. She did amazingly well, and Gib never went hungry.

Gib's children wanted to see their father as much as possible during his odyssey. They felt that his long voyage deprived them and the grandchildren of his company, when they knew there was so little time left. Before he set off they told him that they would visit him on the journey. They also planned to spend a weekend with him when he arrived in New York, which Gib was forecasting would be around the 4th of July.

On Saturday, June 5, Gib pulled up the anchor and moved to the Melbourne Intracoastal Marina, where the twenty-nine-foot *Ka Ching* was dwarfed by opulent fifty- to one-hundred-foot luxury yachts. Around noon, Gib's daughter Lynnea and a friend came to see him. Lynnea soon learned about Gib's special cocktail, the Rum *Ka Ching*, and she and her friend joined him in a little partying.

That evening, Lisa arrived with her son Zack and found that Gib was quite drunk. Lisa was very angry with Lynnea: "What were you thinking about? You know he's sick!" Lisa was only slightly mollified when it became clear what had happened. When Gib was no longer able to take his rum and coke by mouth, he began pouring the Rum *Ka Ching* straight into his PEG tube. What he didn't realize was that in his normal state, before he became unable to swallow because of the ALS, he would drink "a double finger of good rum" in a leisurely fashion over an hour. Now, he was putting two jiggers of rum straight into his stomach in a couple of minutes. This resulted in a rapid rush of alcohol into his bloodstream. When he took a second Rum *Ka Ching* with Lynnea and her friend, he became very drunk.

Lisa and Lynnea put their father to bed and went to a local hotel for the night. The next morning, Gib did not answer his cell phone when they called, and they became very worried. They rushed to the marina and found their father with a doozy of a hangover. Lynnea and Lisa helped Gib to get up and around. He indicated that he needed to go to the ship's chandler to get supplies. They realized that their dad's speech was impossible to understand and went with him to interpret. They worried how he was going to manage when he was on his own again, because his "spit-mumble" speech was no longer intelligible.

In an e-mail to Marcia that evening, Gib told a slightly different version of the story.

From: Gib Peters
To: All my family and friends
Subject: PEG tube

Saw Lynnea and Lisa and Zack last night and today. They held my arms down and poured rum and wine into my tube. I haven't been so drunk in forty years! Before I fell asleep, I had a great time. George expected tomorrow. I'll be in Melbourne till Tuesday, and then onwards.

Love you.
Gib

~~~~~

From: Gib Peters
To: All my family and friends
Subject: Cormorants

The river today was calm, and the sky is clear. Cormorant birds were diving for their breakfast a few hundred yards off the bow, catching and gulping down small mullet. The cormorant is a mostly black aquatic bird with webbed feet, short legs, a dark, elongated body, a long neck, and brightly colored bare patches on its face. It feeds underwater on fish, crustaceans, and other aquatic life, often diving to a hundred feet or more, but not here. I read somewhere that the cormorant is sometimes used by the Chinese to catch fish. A small metal ring is put around its neck so the fish it catches can't pass down the gullet. Clever people, the Chinese.

I subconsciously watched in the silent hope that one would be Gorge, the Water-Walking Wonder of Hawks Channel. I met Gorge, a cormorant, about fourteen years ago when I first began fishing in the Keys. That morning was much like it was today—quiet and bright. I was standing in my little seventeen-foot center-console Mako, anchored about three miles offshore, getting ready to try my luck at catching a couple of yellowtail snapper for dinner. I was unwrapping a frozen five-pound block of chopped-up mullet called chum, which is used to attract fish to the angler's boat. A lone cormorant sailed past, spotted the chum, and circled once before landing on the water about fifty yards away. He ruffled his feathers, settled his wings against his sides, and began a strong, nervous paddle around my boat with neck stretched and eyes bulging. His attention seemed to be riveted to the chum in my hand, but I had other plans for it. I tossed the chum block into a square plastic "egg crate" that had floats on the top and dropped it into the water behind the boat. It floated back on a length of short line tied to the boat and bobbed in the current. Soon, small pieces of fish began to thaw, break off, and sink.

Friend Cormorant was now circling closer, about thirty yards away, with his little black eyes fixed on my fishing rod and reel, head snapping this way and that, as if to say, "Where's the fish? Where's the fish?" Yellowtail snapper is a delicious, light, flaky fish ranging in size up to eighteen inches. Twelve inches is the legal minimum. I baited up, tossed my line into the chum stream, and waited. The flip of my rod triggered the bird to speed up his paddling and move in closer. He was now swimming energetically around in tight circles about ten yards from the transom of my boat, dipping his head under the water to see if any fish were nosing around my bait. Up the head would come: "Where's the fish? Where's the fish?" And down it would go again to catch sight of the school of small yellowtail that was beginning to collect under his feet. This guy doesn't want my chum; he wants my yellowtail!

Well, I hadn't been fishing in Florida long enough to understand the behavior of the fish I was looking for, not to mention the birds that feed on them, but it occurred to me that this behavior was curious, if not remarkable. He was close in and obviously knew exactly what I was doing. It wasn't long before the first fish took my bait. The line went straight and zipped through the water. Friend Cormorant went ballistic, leaping straight up out of the water and flapping noisily toward my boat. Without missing a beat, he landed on the transom next to the outboard motor. He quickly "waddle-turned" around to face the action behind the boat, riveting his attention on the straining line in the water. He extended his wings excitedly to their full length like a miniature Dracula, hopping and bobbing impatiently! "Where's the fish? Where's the fish?"

I tugged my catch out of the water and swung it toward me. It turned out to be a small yellowtail about eight inches long, too small to keep and too big to toss over to Friend Cormorant. After all, Gorge's neck was a skinny inch in diameter and about eight inches long. I was about to toss the fish back into the water but hesitated. "Oh, what the hell, let's see what he does with it." Now, totally consumed with excitement, he fixed his beady eyes on the fish. I tossed it over to him. Not surprisingly, he caught it, did some cormorant "sleight of beak" trick, and down it went head first, still flipping. In amazement, I watched the form of the still-struggling fish bulge its way down his long, skinny neck. Not satisfied, he waddled in place, looking this way and that, seemingly demanding "More fish! More fish!"

"Hmm. Cheeky little devil! And that fish was bigger than he was! This is so unreal! And he wants more! OK, smart guy, let's see if you can handle one more." It wasn't long before I had another bite and swung in another eight-inch yellowtail. This time I had a little trouble getting the hook out of the fish and apparently exceeded the time allowed by Friend Cormorant to accomplish such an elementary task. His patience exhausted, he flapped his way across the three-foot gap separating us and planted himself on my left forearm with the grip of an eagle! "Geez, fella, give me a little slack!" Luckily, the hook came out just as he had made his leap. He grabbed the fish and he did his quick "sleight of beak" maneuver before bulging it down. "Damn, I've never seen anything like this," I thought. "He is not the slightest bit concerned about getting whacked by an angry angler . . . and by the way, that second fish was more than just a little aperitif. How in the world is he getting them in that little body?" By now his toenails were painfully cutting into my arm, but he showed no sign of leaving. I dropped the rod into the bottom of the boat and persuaded him with a little push to get back to his perch on the stern. "Amazing. But look at him now, the little glutton, he seems to have had enough." Gorge the Friendly Cormorant stood quietly on the quarter panel, wings folded, with a dim, faraway look in his eye as if he was considering the need for an Alka-Seltzer.

But he hadn't left by the time the third eight-inch yellowtail was swung aboard, and unfortunately, instinct kicked in. Bright-eyed and wings spread, he made it clear that the fish was his. "OK, you little vulture, here it is!" It slid down with no effort, but that was definitely the last one the little guy was going to take. Together, those fish weighed thirty-five to forty ounces, and the bird didn't weigh much more. With obvious effort, he turned around and flopped back into the water without bothering to spread his wings to balance the maneuver. Splat! Then he slowly paddled his way around behind the boat for ten minutes before he came to life again. Well, more or less. He was ready to go home, apparently. With an explosion of feathers and water, he raised himself up and ran at top takeoff speed over the smooth surface, straight out toward the reef, for fifteen seconds without rising above the surface one inch. Finally, with a perfect imitation of a gooney bird tumble, he splashed into an ignominious ball a quarter mile from where he started. "Forgot to calculate your weight and balance, Captain Gorge!" He made two more attempts to gain enough airspeed, but never made it.

Gorge finally disappeared in a series of runs and tumbles to the reef.

Gorge and I spent two more pleasant afternoons together that year, yellowtailing in Hawk Channel. His third and last visit wasn't for a free meal, though. He had been fishing and diving with his cormorant buddies before I anchored up. When he spotted my boat, he just moseyed over for a friendly visit, fell asleep on my knee for a little while, and then left. I often wonder what happened to little Gorge and what prompted him to be so cozy with humans. It's more likely that someone had patiently trained him to beg for fish. But I'd like to believe that he flew in from China and turned the tables on us humans by getting me to catch fish for him without having to put a ring around my neck. Clever bird.

Gib

~~~~~

From: Gib Peters
To: All my family and friends
Subject: Boat alarms

There are twenty-two audible warnings or alarms aboard *Ka Ching*. They range from the buzzer that says, "Hey, dummy, your ignition is on, but your engine is off," to the fire and smoke detector in the cabin. Among the ones that rank highest on the danger list are the gasoline fume detectors, whose sensors are located fore and aft in the bilge. *Ka Ching* is powered by a pair of Chevy 350-cubic-inch engines and has two one-hundred-gallon gas tanks below the afterdecks.

The day cruise had been uneventful, and the sun was moving into the western sky, promising a beautiful sunset. Time to check out a nice, cozy anchorage behind one of the many islands along this stretch of the ICW. The traffic along this narrow channel resembles a two-lane highway with huge, heavy boats creating wakes that set *Ka Ching* into uncontrolled rolling and pitching, unless taken by a quick quarter turn towards the oncoming rush and an equally quick return to course to avoid collision with the next guy who's plowing up another challenge to my ability to control the boat.

"I can do that too, you turkeys," I grumbled, and moved the throttles from my normal cruising speed of seven knots up to fifteen. My Chevys were now working hard, pushing a very heavy *Ka Ching* through the water and making expensive wakes across the channel for others to admire. I held that speed for about five minutes, until I spotted my anchorage among a group of sailboats and motor yachts in the lee of a mangrove island a quarter mile off my starboard bow and reduced speed again to seven knots.

I had barely completed my turn toward the island when the dreaded sound of the gasoline fume alarm began. Beep, beep . . . then silence. Beep, beep for a moment, then off; but increasingly on, and then continuous. It didn't take more than the first beep for me to have the ignitions turned off and the bilge blowers on, with the windlass free-spinning the anchor to the bottom.

I've always been terrified of that particular alarm after an experience one morning back home in Key West. *Ka Ching* was tied up to my seawall on Riviera Canal, and I ambled out to what I thought was a false alarm to find the bilge fairly sloshing with gasoline. An aluminum gas tank had finally developed a hole, which spilled out some twenty gallons of explosion-producing fumes. I crept off the boat, called the fire department, and they bravely—very bravely—boarded *Ka Ching* to blow out the fumes and start gasoline recovery operations. Obviously *Ka Ching* survived, but the two aluminum tanks were quickly replaced by new custom-built fiberglass models with all-new hosing to the carburetors. Now the nightmare was happening again, far from any firefighting guys or a fast exit to safety.

I shot down the bridge ladder to the afterdeck and nimbly opened the engine compartment to see the devil himself looking up at me from the bilge below: glistening, sloshing liquid about two inches deep flowing back and forth along the keel spar. "Oh God! Think. Think! What are the priorities?" It's only me out here. I've got to think this one through carefully: survival, then protection of the boat, in that order. One spark from anywhere could set off a conflagration and the end of a beautiful idea.

I unlocked the dinghy, cranked it down into the water, and tossed in cat 1 and cat 2. In case of a fire, we could be away in ten seconds. Then I concentrated on air exchange. I carefully opened every hatch and compartment, while exercising a steely determination to be calm and deliberate. That done, I sat on the transom and considered my next move. My crew was fast asleep on the bottom of the dinghy under the outboard.

The first task was to try to determine exactly what I had in the bilge: gas, oil, water, or a combination of all three. If there was any gas whatsoever, it was very bad news. If it was oil on water, I was safe, but challenged to find the source. If dirty water, then what triggered the alarm?

I began to feel a sense of control creep in and mustered the courage to get my face into the bilge to scoop out a sample of the gunk. Did I mention that I am unable to smell? Anything! Not sizzling steaks, salt air, farts, and certainly not gas fumes. A distinct disadvantage on a gas-driven inboard cruiser.

From my flying days, I remembered the routine of draining a bit of fuel from each airplane gas tank into a transparent test-tube-like device in which different liquids would layer themselves, allowing the pilot to see whether there was any water in the gas. Gas floats atop the water. Oil in between. I dug out one of my feeding tube syringes to view the contents of the bilge and discovered a TWO-layer glop: water on the bottom and oil on the top.

"Hey, look guys! Check this out: no gas!" I spluttered through drooling spittle to the cats now sitting wrap-tailed in the dinghy, staring at my face and trying to figure out what the hell I was talking about. The gasoline fume detector was apparently overwhelmed by a large oil discharge and read it as gasoline. Now I had to find the source of the oil leak to see if it was fatal or repairable. It didn't take long to figure out what had happened.

While showing off my enormous speed and wake-making capacity to my counterparts on the ICW, the bow had risen a full eighteen inches over the center of pitch, and the stern had dropped some eight inches below that level. *Ka Ching* was loaded too heavily to move to a level plane and therefore remained in that position for the full five minutes that I was going at full throttle. That allowed the oil in the engine pans to move backward and upward into the dipstick tubes, one of which was sealed—but the other was not. It was the "not" dipstick tube that sputtered oil out into the bilge.

Checking the oil levels in each engine confirmed it. No other sign of an oil leak was obvious, so I just climbed out of the engine compartment, heaved a sigh of relief, and went to find my bottle of Myers Dark. That was the most beautiful sunset I've ever seen.

Love to you all.
Gib

Gib's children wanted to see as much of him as they could while he was traveling through Florida. His daughter Kim went with her husband, George, and their two young children to visit Gib on his boat at the Melbourne marina on June 7. Their daughter,

Lyndsee, was only a few months old, but their son, Dylan, was two years old and was very excited to see grandpa and to chase the kittens around the boat.

The next morning, Gib cast off and continued his cruise up the Intracoastal, arriving at a marina in Titusville, Florida, on June 9. This part of the ICW is up to four miles wide, and the dredged channel runs on the west side, closer to the mainland than the barrier islands. On the eastern side lies the innermost barrier island, Merritt Island. Two bridges link Titusville with Merritt Island; the northern one is a swing bridge, and the southern a cantilever bascule bridge.

Merritt Island is home to the John F. Kennedy Space Center, with its massive buildings that house the shuttles and the gantries that launch them. Rocket launches from Cape Canaveral are spectacular, particularly at night, but there were none when Gib was cruising that area.

Gib's e-mails were reaching an ever-widening circle of friends of friends, and a number of them also had ALS. Many wrote to congratulate him on his courage, and his evenings were increasingly taken up with replying to these responses. The daughter of Gib's friend Mel Fisher was inspired by his e-mails and wished she could ease his pain and suffering. Taffi shared with him her dream of taking a similar long sail, and he wrote the following in reply.

From: Gib Peters
To: Taffi Fisher
Subject: Your e-mail

Wow! How to get to know your friends better: Go to sea with your e-mail machine. I think I have learned more about you from our two e-mail exchanges than ever before. Every thought you shared made me reflect even more deeply than I had allowed myself before. Jerry Cash, Bill Schwessinger, Dick Moody, and countless others secretly (or not so secretly) share the same dream of a long sail. "Just do it," I advised Jerry. "It could be too late tomorrow."

Ronald Reagan was buried today. He faced his Alzheimer's with grace and candor. He said ten years ago that he was beginning a voyage which would lead him into the sunset of his life. It is a simple phrase that appeals to me, and a vision that deserves more than just a place in the book of quotable quotes. It is a description of my voyage.

The trip itself doesn't require courage. It's simply another "controlled adventure." The courage, I suppose, is watching the water and islands pass by and coming to grips with the certain realization that I'm dying. "How does one handle that?" I ask myself. "By denying the urge to just fold in and decay. Finding ways to work around physical problems." Here's one example. My right arm is now weak enough that the weight of a glass of water is almost too much. So I find a place to rest my elbow and challenge the other functioning muscles in my hand and shoulder to take up the slack. Or my faithful but ailing left arm comes flashing in to the rescue! That's victory!

There is no pain, apart from the late-afternoon neck ache caused by the weakening of the neck muscles.

Faith and Hope have become treasures. I'm 90 percent sure that Faith is a lady and Hope is a guy, despite the name. When he's older, I imagine he'll get into a lot of fights because of it. It's a thrill to watch new life. Over the last three weeks they have grown fat, happy, and thoroughly accustomed to the motion and routine of life at sea. At nine weeks old, their world has grown from the aft deck to the cabin (through a flap door in the bulkhead) and the tabletop midships. After days of practice springing, clawing, and thumping back to the deck, now leaping to levels more than four times their length is kid's play. They insist on bounding up to the vee-bunks at lights-out and streaking around together over the blanket, behind the books, and through the rope locker, playing "cat tag and tumble." When the game gets old, they find my feet and curl up for the night. Yesterday, Faith woke up and jumped to the top of the book line for a more advantageous view of the new day. Because of the rocking of the boat, she landed in a spot she didn't plan on and immediately thought she was under attack. So far they haven't quite found the courage to jump up to the after-deck gunnels and parade around the stern and bows, just one slip away from perdition. That's next, I guess.

They're two of the most talented cats afloat. Through careful scientific research and patient observation these last three weeks, I've come to believe that these two have radar. Not the kind a vessel employs for safety at sea, but the kind that tells them exactly what's going on around them. Let me explain my radar thesis. Their world is a twenty-nine-foot-long Wellcraft Sportsbridge with a semicomfortable underbridge cabin that has a three-by-three-foot table midships on the starboard side. The head and galley are on the port side with a pair of vee-bunks forward. The table has two hard-on-the-back bench seats on either side, where I try to make myself comfortable to write and work on small projects. I "eat" standing up because my feeding tube formula goes down faster that way. Mealtime around here is a flat three-and-a-half minutes for both me and the cats.

Now, these cats have the run of the place and can sit any damn place they want, except one: my keyboard, which of course is where they zero in on every chance they get. That was my first clue that they had a conspiracy going or radar that told them exactly where the center of action was. You will remember that with the Windows operating system, if you hold down a key for any period of time, it repeats a series of keystrokes as long as you hold it down. And if it's not a letter or some function or other, a series of "bongs" tells you that you are committing some dumb keyboard error and to get on the right key. If I leave the keyboard for a moment to get a new "spit towel," their radar says: "He's gone. Let's get onto the keyboard and drive him nuts with a few typos and lots of bongs." Zip! There they both are sitting straight and pretty, tails around their little bottoms, smiling at me with sharp pointy ears and pale blue eyes. I can hear them saying: "You lose, turkey. You forgot to close the cover."

So I scat them off and erase the long series of WERTSDF letters from one little offending butt that sat on the left side of the keyboard. But that isn't the conclusive test of radar capability. Being the careful observer that I am, I add this evidence. I needed to do some rewiring of a malfunctioning battery charger behind the vessel's electrical panel. The panel is located at deck level under one of those bench seats and requires a working position not unlike the one taken by a Moslem on a prayer rug. But in my case with a screwdriver in hand. Plop, plop; two tiny furry bodies jump down from wherever they were hiding and stroll over to the worksite. Just watching from a foot or two away is not enough; Noooo! They each vie for position between my straining eyeballs and the now invisible screw I'm trying to remove, offering a helping paw at the point of contact between the screwdriver and the screw.

How do they know that this is precisely the place, within millimeters, where I don't want them? Do they have some sinister conspiracy in mind to piss me off? Nope. I don't think so. They don't talk between themselves very much. It's got to be radar.

How do they know exactly where I am going to sit down? I get up from my rocking chair on the afterdeck to funnel a glass of water into my feeding tube. When I return I find them both curled up on my spot grinning at me. "OK," I say, "I'll use the chair on the port side. You guys keep the rocking chair." Is that good enough for them? Oh, noooo! I get up from the port-side chair to adjust the sun visor, and two tiny bodies streak to the very spot my buns just vacated.

What the hell is this? It's conclusive. Radar.

Warmest regards.
Gib

The old boat *Ka Ching* suffered a number of frustrating equipment breakdowns and failures on the voyage. On June 13, 2004, Gib tied up at the busy Daytona Marina and Boat Works with a broken anchor windlass. He was expecting quick service, but found that it took two days for the replacement part to arrive and another day to complete the repair.

However, the delay had a silver lining because it allowed his son-in-law George to visit him again for dinner and conversation on Sunday night. For Gib, "dinner" meant running three cans of liquid nutrition into his PEG tube, before he and George went to a restaurant so George could have a proper dinner. "Conversation" meant that George talked while Gib nodded and grunted, and occasionally wrote something on his pad.

From: George Cruse
To: Gib Peters
Subject: Thoughts

Been struggling for some time how to express my thoughts about what is happening to you. In reality, this is your final voyage. I understand your love of the sea and have taken many journeys with you. Aside from your blessing to make your daughter my wife and the births of our children, some of my most memorable times have been spent on the water with you. These are things I never had the opportunity to experience with my dad. You accepted me into your family as a son, not a son-in-law. We forged a bond that will forever be a part of my soul, and for that I thank you. When I needed advice, needed an opinion, or just a voice, I could just pick up a phone to call you. That is what I miss most: just hearing your reassuring voice on the other end.

Having something taken from you and not being able to do a damn thing about it is the most difficult and unfair sentence that can be passed. I always try to make something positive out of negative situations. For the life of me, I am unable to do this with your disease. So what do we do? Again, I don't have an answer. Hopefully through an e-mail you can advise me.

Your legacy will live on through your family and your grandchildren. I hope that I can be half the father to my children—your grandchildren—that you have been to your children and to me. It meant a lot to me to see you last week, and dinner last night was wonderful. I didn't realize how much the ALS has robbed you of your strength. There is one thing that is certain: It may rob you of your strength, but it can't rob you of your mind and your will. And now you have started this journey. All I ask is that you make it safely to New York. If I have to carry your ass down Fifth Avenue, so be it! We'll get the boat back to Key West; you just make it to NY!

Love you, Dad.
George

~~~

From: Gib Peters
To: George Cruse
Subject: Thoughts

It's hard to see, I know. But it's OK. I've come to accept it for what it is, and I wish for my family to do so as well. I'm grateful for your ever-ready support and continuing flow of encouragement. With all this support I am able to focus on tomorrow and the day after in my effort to make the most of the time that I have left. Your love is a treasure. You are a son.

Love always.
Dad

~~~~~

Three months later, George sent a follow-up to those thoughts.

From: George Cruse
To: Gib Peters
Subject: Thoughts

As we hunker down for another hurricane, I am finally getting an opportunity to reflect on your previous message and offer a response. These are some of the same thoughts that I felt you were bottling up inside. To some degree we are all waiting for the inevitable. But to have the way you want to live your life, in a sense, taken away from you can be devastating. If you let it! My admiration, respect, and love for you have increased more than I ever imagined. The things I had been searching for earlier in my life, the many mistakes I made, compounded by poor choices, were all righted when you granted me the hand of your daughter Kim. As I thought at the time, that brought completeness to a previously unfulfilled and incomplete life. What I didn't count on was my relationship with her father. Perhaps if I had this inspiration in my earlier years, I wouldn't have made some of the mistakes I made.

But I can't waste time reflecting on what might have been, and must seize the opportunity of every day, living it as though it is my last. One day at a time! It has been very difficult not being able to pick up the phone this last year to get your thoughts on family, business, fishing, whatever.

There comes a time when the teacher has to let the students go to experience life's great journey on their own. It certainly makes my life easier, knowing that for a while at least I have you there. I wish that things were different. But they can't be, so I must apply your teachings and provide for our family in a way that I hope would make you proud. I just want to hear you say: "That's my boy!" So hurry up and complete your journey, be safe, and get your ass home! I still have to learn how to drive that boat so that I can take your grandchildren out fishing, diving, catching bugs, just like their grandpa showed their old man!

I love you.
George

~~~~~

From: Gib Peters
To: George Cruse
Subject: Thoughts

You know, I think this separation from Mom, you, and the rest of our family has sharpened my ability to love and communicate my love to a significant degree over what being within arm's reach could have achieved. Perhaps it has helped us all. I don't imagine that I would have heard such wonderful things from you if we were sitting on a couple of bar stools over beer and wings. But then, maybe so. You are a dear and sensitive guy who continues to amaze me with your manhood and fatherhood. The past is gone. You are who you are, not who you were. We all are. What is certain is that I could not have been able to acknowledge your love verbally from a bar stool. I do so here, and I promise it eternally. You have given my daughter happiness.

I am anxious to teach you all about *Ka Ching* when I return. With a little love and care, she will serve you well.

I love you.
Dad

Since Gib saw Marcia at least once every four weeks when he returned to Miami for the research trial, his e-mail correspondence with her was generally about the mundane, the logistics of getting supplies to Gib, and matters relating to the house in Key West. One constant problem was that Gib kept leaving his cell phone behind at marinas. Marcia would get a call from Gib on a landline and would know what had happened, even though he could not speak clearly enough to tell her. She would then call Gib's cell phone number and speak to the person who had found the phone. She would get it mailed back to her and then send it for Gib to receive at his next port of call.

However, sometimes he let his emotions show through. He would write a postscript to Marcia: "Love you. Thanks for letting me do this!" Perhaps his feelings for his family were best revealed by his frequent anxious e-mails whenever a hurricane threatened

Florida; he was always giving advice on how to avoid the dangers of these storms, several of which hit while he was away.

The e-mail connections that Gib made with his friends of many years, like Wally Dutcher, Bill Schwessinger, Dick Moody, and Jerry Cash, had an intimate and sometimes ribald tone to them. But coming through loud and clear was his friends' concern for Gib's welfare on this dangerous odyssey. Perhaps most surprising was the warmth and intimacy that his e-mails established with his ever-widening circle of e-mail contacts. Some of these were old high school friends. Others were strangers who read his columns about the journey in the *Key West Citizen* or who received his e-mails passed on by friends.

A few of the people who contacted him were patients also suffering from ALS, one of whom had been a classmate at Shorewood High School. Gib wrote: "Must be something in the water of Lake Michigan!"[1]

---

1 Gib may have been closer to the truth than he realized. Recent groundbreaking research into primitive photosynthetic bacteria called cyanobacteria, a frequent source of contamination of our water and food supply, suggests a possible link with ALS. Cyanobacteria are found everywhere in the environment, especially in estuaries, lakes and reservoirs; cyanobacteria blooms also occur in oceans. When you hear of an algal bloom in Florida Bay, the lakes of New Hampshire, or anywhere else in the world, these are usually due to cyanobacteria. For more about ALS, see the Afterword: About ALS.

ib departed from the Daytona marina on June 16 and headed north on the Intracoastal Waterway (ICW). He found a place to anchor behind Fort Matanzas, just off the ICW in the narrows to the western side of Rattlesnake Island.

Fort Matanzas lies on the opposite side of Rattlesnake Island from Gib's anchorage, facing east to the outermost barrier island, Anastasia Island, with the Matanzas Inlet within range of cannon shot to the south. The fort was built on the site of the 1565 Spanish massacre of 250 French Huguenot soldiers who had attempted to attack St. Augustine from the south. After they were captured, the Huguenots refused to give up their Protestant faith to become Catholics, like their captors, who then massacred them. *Matanzas* is the Spanish word for slaughter.

The fort, which has been beautifully restored after falling into disrepair for over a century, is now the center of a small national park and can only be reached by a U.S. National Park Service ferry from Anastasia Island. The fort is small, only fifty feet by fifty feet, with a thirty-foot tower on top. It is built of coquina, a local shellstone, and was first constructed in 1740 by the Spanish to protect the southern approaches to what was then the capital of Spanish Florida, St. Augustine.

The fort is situated fourteen miles south of St. Augustine, which was founded by the Spanish in 1565. Ponce de Leon first sighted the part of the mainland that is now St. Augustine on April 2, 1513. That day was Palm Sunday, or as the Spaniards called it, *Pascua de Florida* or Holy Day of Flowers. He therefore named the peninsula Florida. Ponce de Leon believed that he had discovered the Fountain of Youth in a spring of crystal-clear water near St. Augustine. The spring still exists there and is visited by many thousands each year. No one seems to have found the fountain's magic powers to be any more powerful than they were for Ponce de Leon, who died in 1521 at the age of sixty-one, though that was a ripe old age in those days.

~~~~~

Every night, Gib would find a place to anchor the boat and rest. He wrote about the difficulties of finding a safe anchorage.

From: Gib Peters
To: All my family and friends
Subject: Life at sea

A new sun is burning off the condensation that collected on the outside windows and hull last night, a nearby shoreline is buzzing with bugs and birds, and the pressure is off. I found myself quite nervous last evening when I anchored off Fort Matanzas, south of St. Augustine, because of the brisk five-knot current flowing from the ocean inlet into the tidal waters of the river near the fort.

As always, the decision on when and where to drop anchor is a compromise that balances a number of factors, including fatigue level, channel width, depth, current, traffic, legal restrictions, and whatever. Last night, it became obvious that the current was going to be a major factor. Before long *Ka Ching* was throwing a small, feathered bow wave with a good strain on my "best bower" in the current. (That's how Hornblower would describe his "main anchor." Gotta keep up with the big guys!)

My anchor rode is two hundred feet of half-inch nylon line bent onto a "plow" anchor, which holds well in a mud bottom. But I'm still nervous. If the line parts (very unlikely) or the anchor drags through the mud during the night (quite likely), it would be easy to end up on a shoal downstream. As always, I set the GPS anchor drag alarm, which warns if the vessel moves more than 250 feet from where I dropped the anchor. So fortified, I curled up for a rereading of *The Hunt for Red October.*

Between Ramius's killing of his zampolit and the increasing noise of the river gurgling under my boat, I made a mental check-list of what I would do if the anchor alarm went off. "Scramble to the bridge and start the engines" didn't quite satisfy. So I got up. Better to position the second anchor over the port bow and be ready to drop it first, while I fumbled with the engines. (They can be fussy about being in neutral and having just enough priming to start easily. I'd need the time that a second anchor would provide.) So with the Danforth poised over the rail and secured by a slipknot, I was ready to pop up through the forward hatch and pull the slipknot for a fast anchor fall to the bottom.

"Popping up," by the way, is a euphemism for maneuvering my prone body into a position with uncooperative muscles so that my weakened arms could push the hatch cover up and over. From there I could reach the foredeck and pull the slip knot on the second anchor, if necessary. Elapsed time, about 30 seconds.

Back to the bunk and *Red October.* Ramius gives his pep talk to his crew about their mission through dangerous waters near American imperialist hunter/killer subs. "So, how would I confirm that I'm really adrift?" I ask myself. "Could be that the GPS guys just jinked the satellites a little, and I'd get a false alarm. In the dark, really dark, I'd have no idea, except from the GPS map display, that I was adrift. And that might be a false reading." Out of the bunk again to get the spotlight. Now, with two-million candlepower visual aid at my side, I could "pop up," check the shoreline for movement, and THEN pull the slipknot if needed. Back to the bunk and the book.

"What if, in the dark, I can't find neutral on the transmissions to get a fast start on both engines?" Back to the bridge to set the transmissions to neutral and check the starters.

I felt better. Let the river flow, even roar if it wants to. In fact, I hope it drags. . . . I'd like to see if all my work would pay off. At sunset the tide shifts, *Ka Ching* swings 180 degrees, and begins making gurgling noises with her nose to the west, but she doesn't move away from her tether. Back to bed. Ramius will have to wait until tomorrow night for me to solve his problems. I'm exhausted.

Love,
Gib

Gib remained at Fort Matanzas for a second day. He spent the time catching up with things around the boat.

From: Gib Peters
To: All my family and friends
Subject: It's good to have air-conditioning

I'm writing this morning at my cabin table anchored in Fort Matanzas Inlet, some twenty miles south of St. Augustine, in twenty feet of water surrounded by mirror-flat water and marshy land a few hundred yards away in all directions. It's going to be a hot day; already eighty-two degrees at 7:30 a.m. The generator and air-conditioning are on full blast, basking me in seventy-degree comfort. I'm feeling smug this morning about my decision to install a new five-kilowatt generator to power the 120-volt systems on board, including the AC.

Love,
Gib

The next day, *Ka Ching* cruised past Jacksonville Beach and Atlantic Beach, two small seaside towns with subdivisions and holiday homes for people from Jacksonville. Jacksonville is the largest city in Florida in terms of area, although only fourth largest in population (1.3 million, compared to 2.4 million in Miami-Dade). The Intracoastal becomes narrower from St. Augustine to Jacksonville Beach. North of Fort Matanzas, the trees become noticeably taller as palms and pines are replaced by tall hardwoods. These are the forerunners of the eighty-foot-tall trees that are a striking feature of the scenery along the ICW from Georgia all the way north to Virginia.

The Intracoastal runs some six miles to the east of Jacksonville, but not so far that Gib could miss the two massive cooling towers of the nuclear generating station that lies north of the city. The St. Johns River runs through Jacksonville, and the stretch from there to its outlet into the Atlantic is a busy commercial river. Gib had a hard time avoiding the container ships, tankers, and barges as he crossed to the north side of the St. Johns River and the relative peace of the Intracoastal as it runs northward toward Amelia Island.

Gib anchored near Black Hammock Island, eight miles north and east of Jacksonville, and continued tinkering with things that still needed to be fixed on *Ka Ching*. This area, like many that Gib saw on his odyssey, consists of interconnecting shallow waterways separating low-lying forested islands, some uninhabited and others with a few houses that are easy to reach by boat but very difficult by car.

From: Gib Peters
To: All my family and friends
Subject: Maintenance on the *Ka Ching*

It's dawning over my waterborne encampment about eight miles north of the St. Johns River and Jacksonville, near Black Hammock Island and Sawpit Creek on the ICW. It was a little more difficult to find a suitable anchorage yesterday afternoon, as the channel has become quite narrow with few deep (seven feet plus) channels or fingers. I finally wedged myself between a deep shoreline and red marker 50. It is only 125 feet wide, and I risked a four-and-one-half scope on the anchor. The channel traffic moved passed at moderate speed and had dried up by 5 p.m. because of the building thunder-boomers and lightning strikes to the west.

The character of the scenery and traffic has changed somewhat—many more straight-dredged channels, tall fifty- and seventy-five-foot pines on a closed-in shoreline with brush and hardwoods reaching for sunshine from beneath. I'm reminded of Wisconsin and the straight county highways cut through virgin forest. I'd like to stand in a deep Wisconsin wood again. Quietly. Not stirring a muscle so that I could better hear a complaining black crow in a field a mile away, a buck against a tree somewhere downwind, and a perturbed grey squirrel nearby telling me that I'm not fooling anybody. I miss it.

The configuration of the *Ka Ching* has changed a bit too. Her bridge had a bench seat that served OK for short trips to the reef and return when in Key West, but had by the time I got to Daytona Beach become the source of excruciating nighttime neck and back pain. The strength required to hold an erect position hour after hour has gone. I searched in vain for a way to support my lumbar back and to balance my head on a point. I couldn't find it on the bench seat. So I took it out and replaced it with a single bolt-down captain's chair with arms. I modified it slightly by installing it with a fifteen-degree back-tilt that solved the problem completely. It's now mounted eight inches higher than the bench, which raises my line of vision over a stainless bar ahead, directly to the horizon. I'm also able to swivel left and right for easier visual checks around and behind me, and don't expect now to be surprised by the whistle of an overtaking tug or trawler. A final touch was to attach the GPS to the right chair arm, which puts the buttons and switches always at my fingertips for fast navigational answers. Neat setup! The bench seat is now on the afterdeck, and the second wicker chair is in some landfill near Daytona.

While on the subject of cool, tension-reducing navigation aids, I'll mention that I left Key West with pages of to-do projects that included my "course keeper," so-called by the manufacturer. In true naval tradition, I call it Iron Mike, my autopilot. Mike had developed a case of electronic Alzheimer's and couldn't keep his mind on his job, becoming useless over time. Until I could get time to fix it, I would sit on my bench or chair, with feet up on the helm, skillfully keeping a constant heading with pressure from the bottoms of my feet. But yesterday was the day for "surgery" on Mike.

The problem turned out to be fairly simple and not one of electronics at all. The compass inside Mike drives the electronics to produce a left or right command to the helm motor, depending on the course selected and the vagaries of wind and water. I found that the compass was leaking fluid from a repair I had made a year earlier. The fluid level was down to half, and the circuit board was wet with the light, oily residue. I cleaned the board, but what was I going to fill the compass with? Couldn't be too hard. Water wouldn't mix with oil, or whatever the stuff was remaining in the bowl. I didn't have kerosene, which I once heard worked. So what have I got? WD-40, of course! Marcia's cure for everything that doesn't work right. I squirted in an ounce, and the card began to float freely again. Yep; east is east and west is west! Surgery was a success. I closed the "wound" and remounted the box behind me on the bridge. It works!

So all day yesterday, I reveled in my brilliance and celebrated my resourcefulness by dangling my feet from my nifty tilt-back chair and watching Mike work his ghostly magic on the helm for a dead-straight tour up the ICW. Neat!

Love to all.
Gib

The ALS slowly spread down Gib's spinal cord from the bulbar area of the part of the brain at the back of his head, killing the motor neurons that move the muscles of his neck. Before he started on his voyage, I had seen some weakness of the muscles pulling his head back. Now those muscles were so weak that Gib had difficulty holding up his head for long periods of time while steering the boat. Ever the inventor, Gib constructed a pilot seat to get around the difficulty. His solution—to replace the bench on the flybridge with a pilot's chair that tilted back fifteen degrees—eased the strain on the muscles at the back of his neck and made it easier for him to steer the boat with his feet: another battle won in the rearguard action against ALS.

It was now a month after starting his odyssey, and Gib was settling into something of a routine.

From: Gib Peters
To: All my family and friends
Subject: Onboard routine

My cruise life has taken on a comfortable routine. Major activities have been compartmentalized into particular segments of the day, while tasks within those segments vary enough to challenge and stimulate. My day begins with the scratching and clawing of two small cats working their way up the forty-two-inch wall of drawers and cushions to the top of my vee-bunk. They've decided by their unerring internal clock that it's time to get the old fart out of bed and persuade him to open a fresh can of tuna mush. A painful peek from under my comforter suggests it's barely first light—predawn. I pull the cover over me and groan, "Oh, come on guys, just a half hour more."

But it is not to be. On reaching my level they transform into a pair of tiny lightning bolts flashing over, into, under, and through my private space. The frenetic, morning hide-and-attack game is on. I've tried for a week to put obstacles into their climbing path, but nothing works. Nothing. They find a way. So I uncurl and start the day a bit soured on the world. But maybe ten hours of sleep is enough. Ten hours. I'm sleeping deeply much longer. I don't think it's the ALS, and it's not because I can. I just have to. Otherwise I would find myself dozing in my nifty tilt-back captain's chair and stopping mid-channel somewhere to catch a noon siesta.

So now I'm up, sort of. My three-point pissing position over the head is observed with great fascination by the combatants who by now have called a truce. Hope stretches his full length on short hind legs to peek over the bowl for a better view at the source of the noise. I'm sorely tempted to swing my aim left for just a moment to get even. But I know if I do, I'd add another item to my morning cleanup list. I let the moment pass.

I get my pants hitched up, feed the terrorists, and check for overnight anchor drag. Breakfast is a can of medium-well fillet steak, another can of eggs over medium, with a third can of hot Harpoon Harry's breakfast potatoes on the side. Ah, I wish it were so! Each of three meals a day is the same: twenty-four ounces of a product called Jevity 1.2 Cal, which translates for me into "old-people's food, 285 calories a can." I line up ten cans for the day on the unused galley stove, carefully select three that sound appetizing, and pop the lids. And down they go. My best time so far is two minutes and forty seconds, dictated primarily by the extent to which I remember to relax my diaphragm and stomach muscles. Tomorrow I'm going for 2:30. Blueberry pancakes.

By the way, I've gotten very good at tossing the empty cans into the trash bag about six feet away, over the bilge pump. I'm now working on a left-hand wrist movement that would have them clink together, open-end up, in a neat row on top of my earlier meals. Two out of three ain't bad. God, I'm good.

Gotta go. Sun's up. I've got to cut the first ten feet off a badly chafed anchor rope and re-splice it to the chain. Then it's off to the great state of Georgia about two miles to the north.

Love,
Gib

On Monday, June 21, *Ka Ching* surged northward out of Florida waters and into the Georgia Intracoastal Waterway, near the naval base at Kings Bay. This is one of the many places along the Atlantic Intracoastal Waterway where the sailor finds himself just yards from the shore of a military facility, while motorists can't get within ten miles of the base without being challenged at gatehouses and checkpoints.

Gib's next e-mail and the one he sent the following day were published serially in the *Key West Citizen* as the next four installments of his weekly column.

From: Gib Peters
To: All my family and friends
Subject: Slip and fall

I awoke early this morning to the throb of new bumps and bruises I collected yesterday. While Faith and Hope played cat-tag on the vee-bunk over my sore body, I thought about the events leading to a spectacular pratfall I took on the afterdeck and what it meant about the progress of my ALS. The accident forced me to become a bit more thoughtful about the true condition of my body these days and the subtle changes that are occurring to it as I live out the last of my life. Let me tell you what happened and what I'm thinking.

Maneuvering around *Ka Ching* is easy enough in fair weather, with deck shoes and a good handhold, but the odds of slipping and falling in any boat increase dramatically if any of these conditions is missing. In my case yesterday it was the deck shoes. As the morning formula was going down the tube, I peeked around corners and under the table for them. No joy. I then recalled that I was chased off the afterdeck rocking chair last night by a thunder-boomer downpour and left the shoes behind.

"Yep, there they are under the chair and they're soaked. Well, leave them there and they'll dry by noon." Breakfast finished, I considered an early start up the ICW. So I began stowing equipment left adrift in the cabin last evening to get ready to be under way.

As I emerged from the rear door of the cabin into the muggy air, I searched the horizon for anything new, while reaching up thoughtlessly with my right hand to find the ladder to the bridge. But my right arm was not receiving quite enough brain signals to move itself up to the rail. I grabbed weakly at empty air and was caught a little off balance.

The next few moments went into slow motion. It seemed that I could see what was happening in great detail, anticipate what was going to happen next, and be powerless to stop it. My right foot came out from under my center of gravity. The left never got the signal to replace it, and down I went. Since my neck muscles have all they can do to support the weight of my head when erect, they failed to stiffen as the deck came hurtling up toward me. "Jeez," I thought, "my head just bounced off the deck and here it comes again for another bounce."

Finally, when the slow motion fall came to an end, I was on my back looking up at a swirl of stars framing the little heads of Faith and Hope, who were peering over the bridge deck to see what was holding us up. My ribs, back, arms, and head were new hosts to some ugly bruises. And my sense of confidence was equally bruised. I crept stealthily and carefully around the boat, with wet shoes, for the rest of the day, making sure that I had a grip on two "somethings" with both hands.

I've been testing my right arm over the course of the last two weeks to see if I could see any change in a measure of its strength from day to day or week to week. I think of it as a proxy test for the rest of the muscles. It's a simple test: I try to raise my arm and hand to my right ear, then up over my head with the fingers extended to see if I can touch my left ear. I get there once for every ten attempts. Most of the time I am only able to get my fingertips up to my right ear. On bad days, which are rare so far, I am only able to lift my right arm about halfway to my head.

My muscles are wasting in size all around—shoulders, arms, chest, and legs—and the skin is a bit loose here and there. I've lost forty pounds since the first of the year, but my weight has stabilized at around 170. This was my weight when I married Marcia thirty-eight years ago.

So I think about death. When will it come, how will it come, and will I have a choice to take it on my schedule or will it use its own?

As I cast about for hope and test my faith, I often look to Stephen Hawking. He is probably the most brilliant theoretical physicist since Einstein. I've read two of his books for laymen on the creation and destiny of the universe, but haven't done enough research on the man himself. I think I should. Professor Hawking has been "locked in" by ALS for over twenty years and is a captive of his wheelchair. Yet he still writes! How is it that he has been spared death? Perhaps it's extraordinary medical care he is receiving, or perhaps it is his will to live without the control of his body. Or a lot of each.

I think about death. Hawking thinks about life. My horizon is limited to the time I have left and the lives of my children and grandchildren. His horizon is as deep as the universe and penetrates beyond its known boundaries. I try to reconcile my beliefs about the hereafter. Stephen Hawking ventures into the mind of God. I think he has more to teach me than the fate of the stars.

Love,
Gib

Gib's description of his fall is very typical of what many of my ALS patients have told me. They describe their mind as simply not perceiving their loss of strength. Unless they consciously think about every action, the weakness will catch them unawares, just as it caught Gib and made him fall. Another strange feeling they describe is that on waking in the morning, though they may be totally paralyzed, they feel as if their body has been miraculously cured and they can just get out of bed and walk. Sadly, they learn only too quickly that their mind is playing a trick on them.

Gib described earlier with great pride how he had repaired Iron Mike, his automatic pilot. The repair was excellent, and he had been very pleased with himself, but he was still working out the kinks in Iron Mike.

From: Gib Peters
To: All my family and friends
Subject: Pride Comes Before a Fall

I mentioned earlier that I was able to repair my Benmar Course Setter Automatic Pilot (Iron Mike) by replacing the lost compass fluid with WD-40. It's a two-piece machine; the brain of the system is a box with a compass hidden inside with some electronics, and the other is the brawn of the system with a motor on the helm that turns the wheel when the brain says to do so. I'm thinking of installing a few in my arms and legs next year. Any deviation from the selected course heading will cause a signal from the compass box to turn the motor and the helm right or left. It is uncannily accurate, up to one tenth of a degree in smooth water.

Well, after my brilliant repair job and a few hours of tense observation, I relaxed in my nifty new captain's chair and watched the amazing skill of Iron Mike. He was doing just beautifully, maintaining his course down the middle of a hundred-foot-wide channel to within ten feet of the centerline either way. Fantastic. That tiring steering chore was successfully delegated to Iron Mike, whom I immediately promoted to First Mate ahead of my two other useless crew members, Faith and Hope. Now drunk with power and smug satisfaction, I relaxed with feet up on the console, trusting to a straight shot up a twenty-foot-deep channel in South Georgia.

I haven't seen another vessel of any description for three hours. Hmmm, have I got the right channel? A quick check on my chart plotter confirms that I do. The Garmin Chart Plotter is a moving map connected to a GPS receiver showing my exact position on the globe to within seven feet. Beautifully accurate system. Garmin and old Iron Mike make a splendid pair of navigational tools, which further augments my soaring level of smug self-confidence for this boating thing. Kid's game.

"Alarm, alarm, alarm!!!" . . . then "Karump!" and my engines quit. All within three seconds. I'm aground! Again! How in the hell can that be? I'm too good for this amateur crap! A moment of panic passes and I do a quick assessment. The shallow water alarm went off as I passed over a bar about 150 feet off the center of the channel. A HUNDRED AND FIFTY FEET OFF THE CENTER?! How could I be off so much? And I'm not only in shallow water, I'm in REAL shallow water. Eighteen inches deep at the transom. My draft is thirty-six inches, so my propellers must be buried eighteen inches deep in mud with the tide running. But is it running in or out? Will I sink further into the mud or will I rise free? I hustle around the gunnels, clearing curious cats from underfoot, and attempt to look through the murky water to confirm Garmin's depth warning. I can't see the bottom, but I can see the current streaming around the hull at two knots. And nobody in sight for miles around.

OK, Captain Gib, what now? I don't want to take the time to look up the tide tables to see if I'm in an ebb or flood. But I do remember an ICW guide warning that the tide levels in this area are six to eight feet. Balls of fire, the faster I get off this bar, the better. I formulate a quick plan and release the anchor. I move to the stern and free-fall the dinghy into the water from its perch, and I motor it around to where the *Ka Ching*'s anchor shank protrudes a couple of inches from the surface of the water.

Now I know exactly how shallow the water is. It takes some doing, but I am able to wrestle the anchor into the dinghy. That wasn't as easy as it was a year ago. My arms and back are down to about 30 percent of their pre-ALS strength, but I've got enough left to do the job. I head straight for the channel and deep water as quickly as the little inflatable will take me. The anchor rode pays out from the bow of *Ka Ching*, and at two hundred feet, it snubs. I'm over the channel center and in about fifteen feet of water. So far, so good. I add power against the line and am able to just barely turn the bow of *Ka Ching* toward me, but she won't budge. The tide must be running out. Every minute that passes settles *Ka Ching* further into the mud. No amount of tugging and outboard power are going to pull her free.

Clearly, I'm hard aground. Now what? Nothing to do but drop the anchor into the channel and motor back to *Ka Ching*, now rising like Phoenix out of the water and beginning to take on a very slight starboard list. "No careening here, boat! Your bottom has no sailboat keel, and you should settle into the mud flat and level without tilting one way or the other." Obediently, she does and I'm back on board.

I try Plan B. The anchor is raised and lowered by a powerful motor on a windlass, which can put 700 pounds of pulling pressure on the line and, theoretically, pull me toward the anchor off the mud and into deep water. No such luck. The windlass grinds to a stop without moving *Ka Ching* an inch.

Plan C: Call for pizza delivery! Sorry, that was another time.

A check of the tide table confirms that I'm at dead-low tide. It won't get any shallower than one-and-a-half feet and will begin to flood in about an hour. In three hours I should have two or three feet of new water under me, and the kedge idea should work. I check the Garmin chart plotter to see my track over the last several minutes of travel and see immediately how I managed to end up in the mud. Overconfidence and complacency. Iron Mike did exactly what he was supposed to do and continued steering a straight course, even when the channel turned. I saw the markers ahead but failed to notice that the next marker was a different color, signaling the need to turn! Dumb.

Nothing to do but wait for God's tide to lift me free. So I cleaned house, fed the terrorists, and browsed my library for a good book. *The Black Ship*, by Dudley Pope, looked appealing. Chapter two, and the sun was falling in the west. A huge thunderboomer was rumbling a threat from the south ten miles distant. "THAT could be a complication," I mused. "And there is no way that I'm going to get to an anchorage or a marina before dark." Overcast, no moon, this was going to be interesting and very dark.

A half hour before sunset, I felt a different kind of "bump" from the hull. The tide was beginning to flood and raise my bottom off the mud. "Fantastic!" I tossed the book into the cabin and made my way forward to the windlass. Yes, the line had slackened slightly, signaling that *Ka Ching* had slipped forward over the mud a few inches toward the anchor. I started the windlass and put strain on the anchor chain. I sat on the foredeck and watched for movement by sighting on my errant marker on the channel against a patch of sand on the shoreline. "She moved again!" I mumbled to myself. More windlass strain. "It moved!" I shouted to the cats. "Hey you guys, check this out. She's sliding through the mud toward the channel!" No one else could have understood a word I said through all the spitting and slobbering that accompanies my speech, but they favored me with a moment of spectacular indifference before returning to their cat games.

And so *Ka Ching* slid through the mud until finally she was afloat again. I reeled in the anchor and made a careful dash for the bridge. The engines kicked over and the temperatures remained cool, suggesting that no mud had gotten into the strainers or cooling system. Good to go! Free at last.

But now the hard part. I was twelve miles from Jekyll Island, the only practical next place to anchor or find a slip. My situation had certainly improved, but now I faced a new challenge: navigating to my destination marina in skinny water, long after sunset. Darkness had fallen like a heavy blanket. I checked Garmin for my location in the channel. I considered my new situation: narrow channels, nobody around for miles with local knowledge or advice, and the ever-present problem of my inability to use my radio to explain my predicament. It was 9:40 p.m., and my view from the bridge was like bobbing in an ink bottle with distant green and red fireflies, channel markers, swimming on the horizon. I had a chance of making it if I was bold enough to put on seven knots for good steerage and maintained a dead-straight course up a channel until I reached the next marker. Then the next and the next, until I was out of here. And if I didn't start moving right away, I'd surely drift back onto the mud just fifty feet on either side. And the tide was running strongly already.

Lighted markers are great. But they are generally about a mile apart in this area, and alone are very difficult to use for precision channel navigation. The ranges typically used for this kind of movement are visible only during the day and of no use at night. I formed Plan D, or E, or whatever . . . and decided that if a squall cut off my line of sight to the next marker, I would drop the anchor instantly and wait it out. Did I mention that I hadn't seen another boat for the past seven hours, except for a pair of very fast military boats with tough-looking Seal-types with slung arms, hanging on for the ride of their lives? That was near the Kings Point Naval Station five miles back.

But the next greatest thing to lighted markers and Rum *Ka Ching* is the Garmin chart plotter connected to a GPS. It presents a detailed map of the area, showing my little boat in the center moving over the map. And I wasn't taking my eyes off of it. After all, there was little to see outside the boat save the bobbing fireflies, which are also shown on my Garmin chart plotter with great precision. So I restored Iron Mike to his status as First Mate, glued myself to Garmin's screen, and checked the sonar for depth readings every five seconds. I was flying IFR again! I've said to many of my surprised friends that navigating a boat is far more stressful than flying an airplane. There's little time to correct your mistakes, you're always near the ground, and your passengers tend to want to have another beer and jump overboard to swim with the dolphins. But tonight is a piece of cake. My confidence and my smug are left behind in the mud.

Finally at around 11 p.m., *Ka Ching* and I were alongside a very dark marina on Jekyll Island in Georgia. I idled up to an outside dock, stumbled into some cleats, and tied her up. I gave everybody and everything in sight a kiss. Now it was time to go inside to find my feeding syringe and a tot of rum.

The next morning I was thinking about how my body was doing under the circumstances. ALS is a relentless foe. It kills by inches, destroying the motor nerves that extend from the base of my brain to the voluntary muscles that they control. My tongue was the first part to weaken. Now it's just along for the ride. I can still vocalize but can't make intelligible speech. Before I left Key West, I worried about my inability to use the VHF boat radio, because bridges, marinas, and other boats like to talk before they do business. There are computers available that read in an artificial voice the words you type, but they cost six thousand bucks! I passed. I had found ways to work around the problem by mostly just ignoring the radio altogether or, when really necessary, substituting hand signals, whistles, or just blundering my way through. So far, just "faking it" was working fine. But was I fooling myself?

While I was tinkering with a project on the bridge, I was half-listening to VHF channel 16, the hailing and distress frequency. Suddenly I heard an urgent call for assistance from a fishing charter captain making top speed back to shore with an injured client. He explained to the Coast Guard that a free-jumping barracuda arched into the boat and slashed the fisherman's arm and hand. The captain couldn't stop the bleeding and requested immediate assistance. The Coast Guard was on the scene in about twenty minutes, stopped the bleeding, and took the poor guy off to the hospital. He was lucky.

I turned off the radio and pondered his call and my situation: "What would I do if I was cut and bleeding, or found myself in a situation that required fast communication?" I have a red button on the VHF radio which, when pushed, sends out a coded distress message that includes my latitude and longitude. But it works only if the other guy has equipment capable of reading it. It's a new system and not all Coast Guard stations are equipped yet. And besides, they wouldn't know what was wrong, just that somebody at position so-and-so needs help.

"Well," I mumbled to myself, "my laptop has a couple of tiny speakers that reproduce voice and music, so it just needs software to drive them. I wonder if voice synthesizer software is available on the web." It didn't take long to find the website for ReadPlease, which provides talking software and, would you believe it, at no cost! So I downloaded the program, and bingo, my laptop read exactly what I typed as clearly as a live person could do it. I got it to read its own instructions and Kennedy's inaugural speech. You should hear it cuss!

"OK, you got the computer to talk, Gib; now how do we hook it up to the radio?" That also turned out to be a snap. I connected the shielded audio wires on the remote mike cable to the audio output on my computer through an isolating capacitor, and again it worked. A little distorted and too loud, but understandable. "This is really cool, Gibber. Now let's see if somebody on the other end can understand a typed message." I composed a practice message and turned to channel 16. No one was using the channel at that moment, so I squeezed the push-to-talk button on the mike and at the same time pressed the key on the computer to start reading my script.

"Run Aground Marina, this is motor vessel *Ka Ching*. How do you copy?"

I waited. There was no answer. Of course there wasn't! There is no such marina and never would be. The voice was still too loud, so I turned the computer output down a bit and transmitted my canned message again.

"Run Aground Marina, this is motor vessel *Ka Ching*. How do you copy?" Much better this time, so I began to tape up the wires.

A few seconds later, to my surprise, some guy came on channel 16: "Captain, there ain't no Run Aground Marina inside a hunnert miles of this here river. Go'wan back to New York!"

Fantastic! It works like a charm. I've got speech again. I'm cured! But what was that crack about New York? I listened closely to my computer voice again, and sure enough the voice I had selected—a deep baritone, radio broadcast quality—was really unsuited to the swamps of South Carolina and a working VHF radio. "Probably OK to have this guy read books to me at night," I thought. "But he's got no business on channel 16 in the Deep South. I've got to have a voice that sounds more like a down-home boater. Hah! Check this out," I mumbled to my cats. ReadPlease comes with four voices, two male and two female.

I sent brainwaves to Faith and Hope curled up on the bench seat next to me: "I've just got to do this." They feigned indifference, stretched, and went back to sleep. I selected the silkiest, sexiest female voice available and had her read a new script on channel 16: "Gibby, Gibby, this is Crystal Sue. Can y'all hear me, hon? Ovah." (Yes, the software will actually read accents if you spell everything phonetically.) Ten seconds went by without a response, and then the same guy replied: "Ah, Crystal Sue, this 'ere's Sammy. I hear you, baby. Where you at?" "Gotcha, turkey!" I yelled out at my laptop screen in celebration of another victory over ALS! Whereupon both cats, thoroughly startled, leaped out through the cat door to the safety of the afterdeck rocking chair.

I considered sending the poor guy out twenty miles into the Atlantic to meet Crystal Sue, but thought I was about to step over the ethical boundary into the business of false communications. So, with extraordinary self-control, I pushed the Off switch on the radio and poured another finger of Myers Dark. What a day. Now I can open bridges, make marina reservations, and say bad things to guys who make big wakes. And call the Coast Guard with a meaningful message. And best of all, I can do it as Crystal Sue, queen of the waterways! Life is good.

Gib

Before he embarked on his odyssey, Gib promised to send me updates every few weeks to let me know how he was doing. His messages supplemented his monthly visits to me, which were part of the ALS drug trial. He embellished one of these updates and sent it to his list server.

> **From:** Gib Peters
> **To:** To all my family and friends
> **Subject:** How am I doing?

Some time ago, I told my good friend Doc Bradley that I was planning a single-handed cruise up the East Coast, and he quickly advised me against it. "Why not?" I spluttered. He cautioned that the PEG tube might slip out, that I might fall and have no help around, or that I might choke on something. I got up and showed him my idea of a self-administered Heimlich maneuver over the back of a chair, gesturing back at him: "So what do you think?" He was not impressed. With undisguised irritation, I spluttered back to him: "Never mind, Doc. I'm going!" Marcia rolled her eyes in resignation at my determination and shrugged in his direction as if to say, "What am I to do with him?"

As a final effort, Bradley said to us: "There's new evidence that ALS patients suffer some degradation of judgment. OF JUDGMENT!" he repeated with emphasis to ensure I got the message. My legal training kicked in, and it registered that he was wisely and properly covering himself for any future dumb things I might do up the coast. Resisting the temptation to make the sign of the cross in mock absolution, I mumbled: "Doc, relax. I'm going."

Let me report that in my unbiased, impartial, and objective judgment, he was wrong; my judgment is perfectly sound. Which report, I suppose, is akin to asking a nutcase whether he thinks he's sane enough to walk the streets. After worrying about his admonition and appraising my behavior, I suspect that these "judgment" problems are more the result of miscalculations by

ALS patients about what their bodies can and can't do under rapidly changing conditions rather than of an organic change in the brain. Purely my opinion, of course.

Some of my friends have asked me by e-mail how my ALS is affecting my handling of the trip. Up until now, I've avoided a lot of detail in my answers, but maybe it would be a good idea to report what I see and feel, both for my worried family and friends and for other ALSers who come after me. Isn't that one of my reasons for doing this?

My ALS is the bulbar type, which affects the neurons in the body from the top down; mouth and throat first, then arms, trunk, and finally legs. The rate is variable in different patients, but averages two years from diagnosis to complete paralysis. Motor muscles become weak and finally non-responsive, leaving the mind clear (even Bradley agrees with that generalization). I would describe my present condition in terms of muscle strength on a scale of 5 (normal) to 1 (complete paralysis) as follows: mouth and throat, 2; neck, 3; right arm, 3; left arm, 4; shoulders and back, 4; the rest downward, 5. And my typing fingers still number ten and are going strong.

I'm cheating in my grade of "the rest downward" just a bit. I've noticed changes in my legs during the last couple of weeks. I judge them as "weakening" only because I find it to be necessary to use both arms and some fancy body leveraging to raise my weight (now 175 pounds and holding) to upright from a deep crouch. I am keenly alert for every clue to disease progression and adjust my movements accordingly. Overall I think I'm ahead of the averages at this point, inasmuch as it has been sixteen months since my diagnosis with no apparent degradation in my ability to breathe easily.

The falls have raised my level of caution around the boat to "extreme." Every step on the ever-shifting decks and cabin is an individually prepared, three-point movement: at least one hand on a rail, bulkhead, or ladder for support and two feet firmly planted before moving. I take one step, hold steady, then carefully plan the next. The caution has served me well, and I've avoided many nasty spills as a result. Over the last several weeks, I've found that walking more than a few dozen steps produces a tiring strain on my neck muscles. This is relieved by a simple neck brace on which I rest my chin for longer excursions ashore.

Why do I take the risk? I certainly don't have a death wish. I am not an Evel Knievel nut, but I do, I admit, love risk and the thrill of measuring the odds and validating my judgment. Acting on calculated risk has added zest to my life and coin to my treasure. This cruise is the ultimate test and perhaps the last chance to spice what for me continues to be an adventurous life. So, Doc Bradley, I'm on my way!

Love to all and don't fear for me.
Gib

Ka Ching left Jekyll Island Marina and made her majestic way up the Georgia Intracoastal Waterway without further incident. Gib passed some of the beautiful barrier islands of Georgia, including St. Simons Island and Sea Island, where African American Heritage Sites are home to the Gullah/Geechee culture. The Junkanoo parades in Key West that Gib and Marcia and their friends so loved came from this culture.

In the stretch from Jekyll Island to Savannah, the ICW runs mainly by thickly forested islands and marshes, with little sign of human habitation, other than channel markers and a rare boardwalk running over the marsh from an island cabin. After passing through this beautiful stretch, Gib tied up at Delegal

Creek Marina, about ten miles south of Savannah, on Monday, June 28.

The next morning he awoke to a strange noise coming from *Ka Ching*'s generator that powered all the electrical equipment on the boat, including the air conditioner. The afternoon temperature was in the high nineties, and with the high humidity it felt like 105 degrees Fahrenheit.

Gib decided to have the generator repaired at his next stop, Savannah. On the way into Savannah harbor, he had an encounter that must still be burned on the memories of a couple of old Hispanic gentlemen of that city. He described this in an e-mail that was the next column published in the *Key West Citizen*.

From: Gib Peters
To: All my family and friends
Subject: Sticky situation

You've probably experienced how difficult it can be to pull off a too-small, sweaty T-shirt. If so, you'll love this one.

The summer heat in coastal Georgia is continuous, oppressive, and quite debilitating. The morning air is still, and the reflections of the sun off the water double the power of its radiant heat. Thick cedar and pine stands along the banks block any breeze that might come off the sea a couple of miles to the east. The weather generally is clear to partly cloudy in the morning, until about 2 p.m., when the cumulonimbus begin building for the afternoon downpour. Riding under the control bridge bimini is barely tolerable in the morning hours and all but insufferable in the afternoon. I find that I'm good for only twenty or thirty morning miles a day now because of the heat. Even the big eighteen-inch fan next to me offers little relief.

Yesterday morning I moved from Delegal Marina, south of Savannah, to Thunderbolt Marina in the city itself to see if I could get some work done on my balky generator. Before I started, I pulled out an old black T-shirt that had a Harley-Davidson logo on it. It turned out to be Marcia's damn-near petite shirt size; not the large or extra-large that I wear. "Aw, what the hell. I've lost forty pounds and it's clean. I'll keep it on."

Since I had a feeding tube placed last February, I've been a bit careful about moving around without a shirt because of the danger of snagging the tube on something and popping it out. That would mean a trip to the hospital to have another inserted, and on the Intracoastal that could be quite inconvenient. Besides the safety concerns, a rubber tube protruding from the stomach and clipped to a string necklace to keep it from swinging around causes raised eyebrows. Snug but comfortable with my selected T-shirt, I gave it no more thought but instead concentrated on shifting gallons of drinking water to the bridge for another uncomfortably hot day, as well as planning the route into Savannah. I settled into the bridge chair, fired up the engines, and waved goodbye to the dock master at Delegal.

Perched on the captain's chair, surrounded by canvas and plastic designed to fend off frequent afternoon showers, I felt like a sticky-bun in a hot oven. I poured water down my stomach tube by the quart, which was quite tiring for my weak arms. I considered the feasibility of one of those helmets with a couple of bottles strapped to it and the hoses running into my stomach tube, but discarded the idea. I have however filed it away as an entirely acceptable party trick for back in Key West.

As the early hours burned on, the cumulonimbus began thrusting into the stratosphere to the east. At around noon the gray-bottomed, water-laden clouds moved in for an assault on my little boat moving leisurely to the north. Every afternoon the heat is pushed aside momentarily by the rush of a cool wind dragged down from a high altitude by the heavy shafts of falling water. Then, like the first happy sounds of popcorn in the microwave, the largest drops began to pop, pop, pop on the canvas bimini overhead. And so the afternoon deluge begins.

Rain or shine, my goal was to reach Thunderbolt Marina, about twenty miles ahead. I hoped to find someone to work on my balky generator and was driven by the certain knowledge that where there is no generator, there is no air-conditioning and no good night's sleep.

Along the way, I noted more traffic and turns in the rivers, and a number of small, wooden boats with little five-horsepower motors and grizzled old men drifting the hours away with a pole and line. Each would turn to check me out, wave a friendly sailor-to-sailor greeting, and turn back to his quiet fishing.

By mid-afternoon, the sun and air combined their assault for maximum effect. It was really hot! So I decided to pull off the sweaty shirt before I arrived at Thunderbolt Marina. I rounded a green marker at seven knots and eyeballed the next marker. Couple of hundred yards, I estimated. Enough time.

I steadied the helm on course up the channel and reached over my head with my good left arm for a good tug at the back of the neck of the T-shirt. I got the neck over my head, but immediately realized that this was not going to be quick and easy.

Fifty yards. Hope I'm still in the middle of the channel. The perspiration plastered the shirt to me like sticky flypaper, and I began to feel uneasy about whether I was going to get if off by the next marker. All the tugging and pulling just wasn't work-ing. The shirt wouldn't move up any further. If I had the normal strength in my arms, the shirt would have come off or torn, but my right arm is all but useless and my left is not much better due to the ALS. Wiggling, rubbing, ducking, stretching, and swearing only produced another inch of upward slippage and a tighter wrap.

This was getting scary. Covered now in black from belly to the top of my head, I paused to catch my breath and to offer a small prayer of thanks that I had lost my ability to smell a couple of years before.

Now the top of my head was ringed by the collar of a smelly black shirt and I was virtually blind to the hazards ahead. And it wouldn't come back down again either. I managed a one-eyed peek through the neck to see what I was about to hit. Looking like the black-clad headless Horseman of the Apocalypse, I spied one of those little wooden fishing boats dead ahead at fifty yards with a pair of ancients gesturing excitedly in my direction.

Deciding that the only thing I could do was terminate all effort to remove the shirt and concentrate on avoiding a collision with my fishing buddies, I took a casual position in my bridge chair and spun the helm with my bare feet. With only inches to spare, *Ka Ching* passed the two incredulous old-timers, who now were peering at me with wide, unbelieving eyes.

"Santa Maria," I heard as I glided past. "Es el diablo del mar, Manuel!" "Dios mio, vamonos, Toni." Moments later I heard a flurry of banging oars and the sound of a small outboard fading astern. I turned back to the neck hole to settle on my new course for the next marker. That done, I retrieved my pocketknife and began some quick underway tailoring on Marcia's little, teeny-weeny T-shirt.

I don't know what story those two old fellows told when they got back to shore, but I do know with a high level of certainty that as far as shirts go, it's going to be white and extra-large from now on.

Love to everyone.
Gib

When I read this, I almost fell off my chair laughing—until I focused on the comment about his weakening arms. If he was already having difficulty holding up a bottle of water to pour it into his PEG tube, was he going to be able to feed himself without help for the next three or more months and finish his solo odyssey?

G ib needed to bring *Ka Ching* into dock in Savannah to get his noisy generator fixed. He was afraid that it would break down completely and leave him without power for the auxiliary systems, especially the air-conditioning. The first place he stopped was Thunderbolt Marina, where the folks told him that they were not agents for Westerbeke Corporation, the makers of his generator, but that Sea Ray Marina, just up the river, would be able to look after him. Little did he realize this was just the beginning of the most frustrating three weeks of his life. Gib eventually wrote up his unfortunate experiences as a column in the *Key West Citizen*.

IF YOU DON'T LIKE TO HEAR A GROWN MAN CRY, SKIP THIS ONE!
By Gib Peters

Almost three weeks ago, Tuesday, June 29, I awoke to a new sound coming from my generator. This produces normal house voltage for my A/C, computer, battery chargers, and miscellaneous other appliances and tools aboard Ka Ching. It was the loss of the A/C that worried me the most. I was coming close to the time when I would benefit from a nighttime BiPAP machine to help my breathing. Fortunately a major urban area was just ahead, since finding capable repair services and parts on the ICW can be tough. In this Georgia summer heat I find that running the air-conditioning is the only way to sleep, especially with so many bugs and mosquitoes banging into the sides of the boat trying to get in.

The generator was new in February, and after I installed it into the bottom of Ka Ching, I cranked it for the first time. It wouldn't catch and run, so I fiddled with fuel, checked the ignition, and cranked it again, and again. Finally it "caught" and ran, however now with a "clank" on every revolution from somewhere inside.

I took the boat and generator over to the local Oceanside Marina in Key West to find Mark, the Westerbeke Corporation dealer who sold it to me. He started the engine, listened to the clank, stroked his chin, and asked about how I attempted to start it after installation. I told him, and he guessed correctly that seawater had backed up into the cylinders from the cooling system because it didn't have the pressure of the exhaust from a running engine to push it out. I had "over-cranked" it. As a result, the piston tried to compress the water in the cylinder, couldn't do it. Excessive pressure on the piston rod bent it, causing it to hit the cam shaft sharply on each rotation. He also noted that the warranty specifically excluded seawater damage. So I was condemned to pay for the repairs.

I had the choice of having it fixed by someone else or doing it myself. I've replaced both of my boat's propulsion engines using rebuilt Chevrolet, eight-cylinder, 350-cubic-inch "long blocks," so how hard can a little generator engine be? Mark offered me his workshop and advice if I wanted to strip it down and put it back together with a few new parts. "No big deal," he said. Neat *guy. He knew I was aching inside because of my dumb mistake of over-cranking the generator and that I was trying to make ends meet for my trip up the ICW.*

The short story is that I opened the engine, replaced a bent rod, and closed it up again. It actually ran! Beautifully quiet and smooth. So back into Ka Ching it went, and I took off on my trip.

So three weeks ago I found myself groping around in the early morning, wondering where the clicking was coming from. I made a quick diagnosis that something was loose inside the engine. Remembering the sweat and labor that went into rebuilding the generator when there was salt-water damage, I decided to find a Westerbeke dealer near Savannah, twenty miles ahead, to have it diagnosed and repaired, especially now that everything was under warranty.

The narrow channel soon became a busy harbor dotted with small commercial vessels of every description moving busily about. I dodged under a bridge, around some tugs, and got out of the way of a long sightless barge bearing down the center of the channel behind me. I threaded my way into the upper reaches of the Wilmington River, nearer the city, where small pleasure boats dominated the waterway. I picked a marina that looked like it had some mechanical services. I didn't expect that this particular marina would be a Westerbeke generator authorized repair facility, but I did expect that they could help me find one in Savannah. And they did. After calling around, the dock master pointed up the river and said that I would find my generator repair guys at Sea Ray Marina, just around the bend and under the bridge. "GREAT NEWS," I thought. "They'll be able to diagnose the problem and fix it in a day or two, and I'll be on my way." I scribbled a "thank you" on my clipboard and climbed back aboard Ka Ching. The dock master cast off my lines, and I plowed my way another mile or so up the river.

I eased Ka Ching *up to the fuel dock of Sea Ray Marina, where a couple of young dockhands watched me put my port side to. Hands on their hips, they made it clear that they wanted to know my business before they tied me up. In turn, I made it clear by pantomime that I had to write my request and wasn't able to shout my needs across the water to the dock. They reluctantly reached for my lines and held them unenthusiastically while I dismounted the bridge and scribbled my need for a Westerbeke mechanic because I had a problem with my generator. "We ain't no Westerbeke dealer, mister," the fat one announced. "But I was told you were," I scribbled. "Who told you that?" I pointed to my chart showing the marina a mile back down the river. "They don't know what they're talking about," with a grin back to the skinny guy.*

Back to the clipboard. "Look, I've got a serious problem here. Please check with the repair shop and make sure. OK?" The skinny kid took that as his cue that this was not going to be a fast fueling and would require that he loop my lines around a couple of cleats. After tying Ka Ching *up, he followed me inside. "Heavy" spoke on the phone for a few moments and reported: "Like I told you, we are not a Westerbeke dealer and don't do warranty work for them. But we can look at your generator next month and do the work at regular rates." "Next month? In August?" It was July 1st.*

I was incredulous and growing more than a little irritated with their attitude, and feeling that they were trying to avoid the factory warranty rate schedule. "OK. Who else in town is a Westerbeke dealer?" "Skinny" lifted his chin to the marina across the river about two hundred yards away. "Try them." I angrily climbed aboard Ka Ching, *pushing between a couple of curious cats who wanted to know what was going on. Before I got the engines going, my dock lines, both fore and aft, came snaking through the air and plopped onto the decks. Surprised, I quickly fumbled with the* ignitions and after a couple of anxious moments and a ten-foot drift into the river current, got the engines turning. JERKS!

I had Ka Ching *do her best snotty little pirouette in Sea Ray's approaches and purr herself across the river to Hinckley Yacht Sales, where a young man reached for my lines, tied me up securely, and greeted me with: "How can we help you, Captain?" After a series of hasty, illegible notes from me and patient verbal responses from him, I discovered that the outfit I had just left across the river was, indeed, a Westerbeke dealer and that the Hinckley outfit, where I now found myself, was not. I took a deep breath to see if it would help take the edge off my frustration and listened to the young man think aloud about my problem. "Hmmm. Let's do this," he said. "I'll call Westerbeke and see if they will authorize my guys to do the repairs under warranty. OK?" "I'll be grateful," I scribbled, and followed him off the dock to the office. He disappeared for a moment behind a cubicle divider and then re-emerged, saying: "No answer, but I left a message. Captain, why don't you make yourself comfortable for the night and we'll work something out in the morning?" It was 4:30 in the afternoon and I had used up my store of patience for the day. Seemed like a good idea. I made my way back down the dock while casting inaudible curses and evil spells at the marina across the river, but somewhat hopeful about the young service manager at Hinckley.*

As I approached Ka Ching, *now pitching alongside the outermost dock, I heard an irritated series of staccato "quacks" from the end of the dock. A hundred feet away, a plump female mallard duck was waddling purposefully in my direction, while doing a friendly, submissive low head-wag and making chuckling noises in my direction. I was intrigued and waited to see how this would play out. When she reached my feet, she looked straight up at me and waited. I interpreted all this as: "OK, pal. You tied up* on my dock. It's going to cost you!" It was my turn, I guessed. "Duck food, eh? Afraid it's going to be cat food, Aflac."

Hope and Faith did not seem to mind my digging into their dry food bag. They were too preoccupied with their analysis of the oversize bird on the dock and the raucous new sounds that it generated. Before long there were introductions all round, food and drink for everybody, and a consensus among us that when Aflac was happy, everybody was happy. Maybe this indicated that my situation with the generator would smooth out after all.

I didn't know it then, but the next day was the first of nineteen days at Hinckley's, feeding cats and ducks, writing e-mails to whomever would listen to my laments, and pestering the service manager at Hinckley for word that Westerbeke would authorize repairs. Nineteen days!

The very kind mechanic at Hinckley Yacht Sales did his best to get permission from Westerbeke to look at my generator by faxing a form Application for Warranty Service to the Westerbeke regional distributor, Engines1, in Portsmouth, Virginia. It took Engines1 a few days to read it and suggest that the mechanic look at it to see if he could determine the problem. The mechanic looked and responded to Engines1: "I dunno." It took yet another couple of days for Engines1 to say, "Well, try this . . ." Then another couple of days, and so on. Finally after fourteen days of miscommunication, untrained electricians and mechanics, and wrong parts being sent by Engines1, I called a stop to it.

I was beside myself with frustration. Had I been able to speak, I would have been on the phone from sunrise to sunset until I got action on my warranty. But, then and there, for the first time I discovered the true limits of my speech disability. My e-mails to Westerbeke were ignored, save for the admonition to stay where I was and they would get back to me. As I told my daughter Lisa, it felt like someone had tied my hands behind my back, put duct tape over my mouth, turned a steady drip of water onto my forehead, and could be heard laughing at me from a distance. "*Let's see how pissed off we can get him*" is what I made of it all. I can report that I was HIGHLY pissed and ready to rip a new aperture for the guy in charge at Engines1.

Nineteen days! I had to try something else. I e-mailed Bobby Highsmith, my stalwart Key West attorney, who warned me that legal action wouldn't get my generator repaired any time soon, but that an aggressive, immediate public relations effort might! "*Either way*," he said, "*I'll buy you a new generator and you can be on your way.*" I wondered if he knew that my generator had a $6,000 tag on it, but in any case I declined. This was a matter of principle, not money.

Now I was at the edge of depression. How the hell could I carry out that kind of campaign when I couldn't talk? Then an idea. I turned to my e-mail list of thirty-five or forty good friends in Key West and sent them a copy of Bobby's message to me, with a call to them for help. And what a job they did! The following day, Friday at 4 p.m., a TV crew from the local Savannah ABC affiliate showed up on the dock to see what the generator fuss was all about. It seemed that a dozen or more angry Key Westers had phoned Westerbeke corporate headquarters sharing their incisive views of Westerbeke services, and Madeleine Burnside had called the local TV action line, who visualized the sorry picture of the treatment ol' Gibber with Lou Gehrig's disease was getting at the hands of some big bad corporate manufacturer. The ABC reporter who came to do the interview was drooling after the story, and it was a toss-up whether he or I was drooling more! They shot lots of footage and aired it that night for all of East Georgia to see.

On Saturday morning, the Hinckley service manager came bouncing down the dock, rapped on the hull of Ka Ching, and reported that Westerbeke was sending a new generator and a *mechanic from Atlanta the next day! Sure enough, on Sunday evening around 6 p.m., I heard another rap on the hull. "Are you Mr. Peters, sir?" "Yesshh," I drooled in surprise. He genuflected a couple of times, stammered his apologies for the late hour, and reported: "I'm from Westerbeke with a new generator for you. Could I get started right away?" "Hew, yesshh!" I spluttered. And that's what he did. Before nightfall he had got the old generator loose, and the next morning he and a couple of helpers arrived with a spanking new red generator in a cart. They hoisted the old generator out and the new one in. By Monday noon they had the job finished.*

Perched again in my lofty captain's chair, I wended my way thoughtfully out of Savannah, GA. I resolved to figure out a way to communicate over the phone before I got into trouble with another reluctant vendor . . . but then again, with friends like mine, who needs it?

Life is good!

Gib

The people at Hinckley Yacht Services were wonderful to Gib and never even charged him docking fees. Dustin Hartley, the service manager at Hinckley, tried to get Westerbeke to provide the technical support that his engineers needed. Dustin called and e-mailed Westerbeke many times with no effective response. Despite the difficulty that Gib had in communicating, Dustin and the office manager, Nancy Veenstra, took a great liking to this single-handed spluttering sailor. Dustin and Nancy were filled with the sort of charity that I was thinking about when I suggested the names of Faith and Hope for Gib's two kittens.

Dustin was in his early thirties and had spent seven years in the Coast Guard out of Key West. He and Gib exchanged many stories about the southernmost city in the United States. Tall, fair-haired, bronzed, and handsome, Dustin had left the Coast Guard to captain a seventy-foot private yacht around the Mediterranean and Western Europe. When it was time to settle down, he came back to his hometown of Savannah and started work at Hinckley Yacht Services. During the nineteen days that Gib was suffering through his Westerbeke experience in Savannah, Dustin developed a close bond with this speechless sailor.

A week after Gib arrived at the Hinckley yard, he flew down to Miami to see me for a follow-up examination as part of the drug research study. I saw some deterioration in the strength of his muscles and told him I was amazed that he could manage *Ka Ching* single-handed. He had lost another eight pounds, despite increasing his feeds to ten cans of Ensure a day; I increased his daily intake to twelve cans. Because Gib's stay in Savannah was much longer than expected, Marcia had already sent the next load of "liquid meals" to a marina further north. She had to rush an emergency supply to the Hinckley boatyard to prevent Gib from starving to death.

Gib did not take advantage of the prolonged stay at the Hinckley yard to see the beautiful old town of Savannah, with its wide streets bordered by tall hardwoods draped in Spanish moss, and the medians resplendent with brightly colored flowering trees. He never took a delightful horse-drawn carriage ride that introduces visitors to the historic parts of Savannah, its antebellum mansions, and its two-hundred-year-old parks and monuments. All Gib experienced in Savannah were unremitting heat and humidity, and uncertainty about whether Westerbeke would ever repair his generator.

Following the success of the PR campaign waged by his friends in Key West, he had his new generator, and on July 20, 2004, was finally on his way again, with New York as his next goal. Gib had lost three weeks and worried about the effect this would have on his plans for the voyage. He consulted a number of friends, people who were experienced sailors of small boats, concerning the Great Loop circumnavigation of the eastern United States. Some urged him to "go for it," not knowing his physical condition. Others recommended caution, pointing out that he must consider the effect of bad weather and ice on the Great Lakes. Gib did not ask my opinion, but I would have told him that he would not survive to complete the Great Loop.

To try to make up for lost time, Gib decided that he needed to pick up the pace. He still did not want to push *Ka Ching* to more than seven knots because of his earlier experience of getting oil into the bilge and because of the cost of the higher fuel consumption that would result. He therefore traveled more hours each day and took fewer rest days.

The first night out of Savannah, July 21, 2004, he anchored off Hilton Head Island, at the southern tip of South Carolina. It's one of the largest barrier islands off the East Coast and home to many elegant resorts and fine restaurants. But Gib did not have time to be a tourist. He "ate" on the boat and headed out early the next day, taking a shortcut in the open Atlantic, which, fortunately, was flat calm at the time. He anchored that night ten miles north of Charleston, South Carolina. Again, he did not tarry to visit the historic old city of Charleston, with its attractive waterfront, its antebellum homes, and the fourth-oldest Jewish congregation in the continental United States. Instead, he rushed on, and by the evening of July 25 was anchored just off the Intracoastal, near Cape Fear, at the southern tip of North Carolina. This area of the Atlantic is famous for its treacherous currents and was given its name in the sixteenth century by sailors who narrowly missed wrecking on the Cape.

The morning of July 27 saw Gib cruising northward past Snead's Ferry, North Carolina. In colonial times this small town at the northern tip of another of the barrier islands, Topsail Island, was the site of a rope ferry across the New River estuary. This ferry was an important postal link on the route between Virginia and South Carolina during the Revolutionary War, and the town took its name from Robert Snead, who purchased the ferry in 1760. It is now the home of an important shrimp boat fleet and game fishing charter industry. The town is also known for its recreational and commercial scuba diving for spiny lobsters, which the locals will assure you run up to three feet long and thirty pounds in weight.

North of Snead's Ferry is the New River estuary and Camp Lejeune, the main base of the U.S. Marine Corps. Gib cruised within a dozen yards of the camp, though a landlubber motorist is not allowed within five miles of the base, the road being blocked by barricades and armed guards. As Gib crossed the New River estuary, piloting *Ka Ching* with his feet, he experienced one of the amazing adventures that seemed to happen only to him.

From: Gib Peters
To: All my family and friends
Subject: Memories are the roses of December

I spent yesterday in a do-it-yourself boatyard replacing a starter on the port engine, adjusting throttle linkages, and fine-tuning Iron Mike, my autopilot. This morning, I'm under way again, on the ICW in North Carolina about twenty miles north of Wilmington.

Camp Lejeune was ahead a few miles, but it wasn't clear from my nautical charts exactly where the camp border was. I was soon to find out. *Ka Ching* was moving north at a leisurely seven knots in a narrow channel, when ahead and coming south, no fewer than five orange and gray inflatables came bearing down on me at high speed. They decelerated sharply abreast of me, revealing in large black letters on the tubes: "United States Coast Guard" and "United States Navy."

But what really jarred me were the twenty heavily armed military machos in green camo staring at my vessel. On the "cut-throat" signal from what I would guess was the senior guy, I shifted into neutral and drifted to a near-stop. While I fumbled with the gear shift, I rehearsed my explanation. "OK, guys, I surrender. I admit that I'm carrying two whiskered terrorists on board, but I don't think they are big enough yet to be a security threat." As I stabilized my drift, I thought: "OK, Gibber, let's get serious. Did I forget to switch the head discharge from 'sea' to 'tank' last time I used it? That must be it. That would certainly require twenty burly guys with machine guns to bring my errant behavior under control!"

I ease my way down the ladder to be better able to hear what the charges against me were. "Sir, are you aware that you are in a restricted area, sir?" Hmm, two "sirs" in one sentence. They must be Marines. I do my pantomime indicating that I am unable to speak, but that I can hear OK. That initially bewilders them, but eventually they catch on. Initially they try to return the pantomime, until I point to my ear again and give them the "OK" sign.

"Ah, you are able to hear. Roger that, sir," the PO says. "Sir, the Navy and Coast Guard are about to conduct firing exercises off the coast and over the ICW immediately ahead. You are requested to hold your position here until noon, sir." I consider the quiet vigilance of the other nineteen guys arrayed around me and cheerfully nod agreement with the "request." After climbing back up the ladder, I maneuver to the center of the channel and drop the anchor. The Coast Guard takes off past me to intercept more trespassers, while the Navy anchors nearby to make sure that I don't do anything stupid.

And they weren't kidding.

At 10 a.m sharp, from an unseen warship beyond the mangroves toward the sea rolled a series of sharp concussions. Bang! Bang! Bang! Bang! Bang! Each report followed almost instantly by the scream of a live projectile ripping the still air one thousand feet over my bow. For the next two hours, from the phantom vessel anchored fifteen miles to the east, the guns continued firing. With keen interest I checked the charts for clues as to where the guy could be and what he could be shooting at. I saw that the firing range extends from a square "restricted area" offshore, inland over the ICW to a line about thirty miles inland to the west. Each projectile they fired traveled a long arc and hit its target a full ten seconds later with a muffled boom, boom, boom, mirroring the cadence of the original fire.

Hope and Faith were not at all happy with this rude intrusion upon their leisure. On the first fusillade, Hope jumped a foot straight up off the deck. But because of the easy roll of the boat, he didn't come down exactly in the place he expected. When he got all fours down again, he launched himself off the afterdeck through the cat flap and into the vee-bunk, with his little claws desperately scratching for purchase on the gel coat of the deck at every turn. Faith, noticing the rattled psyche of her brother, thought it was a good time to press the advantage with a new game of attack and wrestle.

Exciting stuff. I listened intently on my VHF to the blue water Navy coordinating their firing exercises. I also heard, but couldn't see, helicopters and landing craft on the beach nearby. Damn, I wished I had a tuna tower over the bridge; I might have been able to see over the top of the mangroves and watch the war games. But I didn't, so I slumped in my captain's chair, sorting through a flood of memories of fifty years ago during my time in the Navy that were triggered by the firing. I could easily smell the burnt cordite again and hear the ring of the expended shell cases being ejected from the breech. Funny how sharp the memories are, even today. Klaxons, fuel oil, Morse code, boson's whistles, sea spray, compass repeaters, radar fixes, bug juice, and shit-on-a-shingle. The pictures flash by so clearly that I'm left to wonder at the power of the human memory.

The Navy was good to me. I have to report that fact honestly, even though they fired me after serving honorably some twenty-three years in the Navy Reserve. When Dutch and I joined the reserves in 1953, we both proudly pulled on our sailors' jumpers that were without insignia, spiffed up the rest of our uniforms, and headed off to the Naval Reserve Center on Milwaukee's lakefront. There we would learn how to talk sailor talk, watch movies about the Tyranny of Communism and Venereal Disease, and listen to lectures about saluting officers. "And if you are passing in close proximity to a commissioned officer, you salute and hold it until it is returned!" droned the instructor. "What do I do if he doesn't return it?" I wondered sarcastically but didn't ask. "And you don't salute a civilian unless he is personally known to you as a commissioned officer. But don't expect a return salute!"

Having absorbed all I could stomach of training films and military courtesy, I was threading my way down a hallway between classes and stopped to check the bulletin board for new correspondence course offerings. My eye caught a small one-inch sentence buried in a thumb-tacked newsletter saying: "New reserve enlistments who are FCC-licensed radio amateurs may be advanced immediately to the pay grade of E-3, Seaman." Whoooa! I got my ham license when I was fifteen, and I certainly was newly enlisted! I carefully pulled out the tack and replaced it at the end of a neat military row of other unused tacks at the top of the corkboard. A closer look at the tiny stand-alone sentence didn't change my first reading. Yep, that's what it says. Anxious to employ a newly learned phrase, I thought, "Let's see if this is the 'straight skinny.'"

The khaki uniform with a ruddy, sea-worn complexion sitting behind the first desk in the Admin Office squinted up at me and said, "Lemme see it, Peters." Startled that this might be another "short arm" inspection, I stammered, "S-see what, Sir?" His squint turned to a scowl. "I am not a commissioned officer, sailor. I am a chief petty officer and I'll thank you to imprint these 'ere fouled anchors onto the inside of your forehead!" "I—" "And you will address me as "Chief." "Yes sir, Chief," I stammered. He took a deep breath, rolled his eyes but mercifully went on: "Let's see your FCC license, Buttkit!" I fumbled for my wallet, finally remembering that it was folded in half over my waistband, and pulled out the little tattered form. "Hmm. OK! Fill out this form, Peters, in triplicate, sign it, and hand it back to me before you leave today. In the meantime, go down to the ship's store and draw a set of seaman's stripes. Now, get out'a here." Holy Fright! I'm a seaman! Three stripes! Whoooo haaa! I outrank Dutch! I gotta go find him and bust his ass!

Where did all that come from? What triggered these long forgotten moments? I knew, of course, but still marveled at the sudden and unexpected clarity of each recalled scene.

I switched back to channel 16 on the VHF and swiveled the chair so I could reach for my Walkman. The earphones masked some of the noise of firing and flooded my head with the steady hissing of background noise before I began the search through the FM band sinkholes and muck for a nearby PBS station. Whoa!

What's this? The Beach Boys are harmonizing a long-forgotten tune called "Barbara-Ann." It isn't National Public Radio but instead one of those "nostalgia" stations for old farts.

I pause and listen for a moment. "Take a chance," they croak. And here come the memories again. They take me back to the dark, smoky bar in the Cuba Club in Madison, Wisconsin, jammed with a boisterous college crowd, where I first met my bride, Marcia. The only light is coming from the dozen neon beer signs. I snag a cold Schlitz out of the ice bucket strategically positioned at the center of the table I am sharing with my two law-student buddies. They hooked up with a pharmaceutical rep they knew and invited him over to the table.

Bad move. The guy drank our beer and complained about his unappreciative girlfriend for the next half hour. His appetite for Schlitz beer was matched only by his size: six-four, two-twenty, a superman shape. I figured he could drink all he wanted.

My attention wandered to the women in the room. I locked onto a petite, perfectly sculpted girl, who was talking animatedly to some friends at the bar. She wore a simple pink and white dress with chestnut-brown hair brushed back to a pair of clips before falling to her shoulders. She looked like a windblown fashion model by the best Fifth Avenue photographers, without the benefit of a fan. Her doe eyes were positively gorgeous. I'm dumbstruck. "She's it. She's the one." I'm instantly deeply in love, and my practiced self-confidence plunges to absolute zero. The drug rep at my elbow is filling my ear with hospital jokes, and the Beach Boys implore anyone who is listening to "take a chance."

Fixated on my new vision, I lean over to the drug rep's ear and ask him: "Who's that girl at the table over there? That's the girl I am going to marry."

"Where?" he asks.

"Right there, on that center stool." I nod in her direction and ask my craning drinking buddies, "Who is she?" The pharmaceutical rep takes a quick look and retorts, "Her name is Marcia and she's my girlfriend, you dink!" I'm oblivious to his irritation and continue staring stupidly in her direction. "Barbara, Barbara," the Beach Boys chant. My competitor's imposing size suggests caution, but I am attracted beyond words. On the other hand, her power to say "no" all but incapacitates me. "Take a chance," the Beach Boys shout again. I do. With rubbery legs I maneuver for the approach, feeling as if my very life is at risk.

The same Beach Boys song that was playing then is playing now, urging me to "take a chance." I did the last time, and the rest is history.

Bang! Bang! Bang! The firing continues. But the mystery of memory occupies me again. Why is music such a powerful image stimulator? Ever notice? Music, it seems, is the primal memory creator; the first to excite, the last to fade. Every note and phrase hits deeply as if they were once connected to an important life event. I find myself in exactly the place where I was when I first heard that tune, recalling every detail, every smell, every note. It seems that memories are at the top of all that is important these days.

The Navy kids break the interlude by reading an "all clear" script on channel 16, giving the queue of idle ICW boats permission to hoist anchor and get under way. Since I was first in line, I quickly winched up the anchor, promoted myself to the temporary rank of commodore, and led the convoy north through the newly won battleground, richer and happier than when the day began.

Gib

It rained all day on July 28, but Gib was warm and dry in the minicabin formed by the bimini and the vinyl roll-down windows around the flybridge. The two kittens sat on the control panel on either side of the steering wheel, watching the scenery and boats go by. That evening, he reached Beaufort, North Carolina, a historic port just east of Morehead City. For the next week, *Ka Ching* traveled through the Pamlico and Albemarle Sounds in North Carolina.

The first violent storm of the 2004 season, Hurricane Alex, brushed the Carolinas on August 4. As luck would have it, Gib was without cell phone coverage in this area and therefore unable to make e-mail contact with Marcia, his family, and friends. The prolonged hiatus in communication made all of us think that something terrible must have happened to Gib in the hurricane. A couple of days later, Gib reached an area where his cell phone worked again, and he sent word that he had been safely tied up in Elizabeth City, North Carolina, when Hurricane Alex blew through.

The 2004 hurricane season was one of the busiest on record for the Atlantic coast of the United States, exceeded only by the record-breaking 2005 season, which included Hurricane Katrina's destruction of New Orleans. In 2004, the Atlantic Basin had fifteen named tropical storms and nine hurricanes, of which six were Category 3 or higher, and five hit the United States. Hurricanes Charlie, Frances, Jeanne, and Ivan all initially threatened Key West. Eventually, Charlie destroyed Punta Gorda, on the west coast of Florida, while Francis and Jeanne both hit Fort Pierce on Florida's east coast. The Peters' home in Key West suffered wind and water damage in several storms, as did their children's homes in Orlando.

Gib felt lucky to be out of Florida but worried about Marcia and their children. Marcia in particular suffered a great deal of stress at this time, not only contending with the storms but also trying to cope with the fact that her husband and lover was dying, the logistics of keeping Gib's food and other supplies coming, and the need to keep her home nursing agency going, since this was now the only source of revenue to cover the cost of Gib's odyssey.

~~~~~

From: Gib Peters
To: All my family and friends
Subject: Accident in the Great Dismal Swamp

The Great Dismal Swamp covers a broad 111,000 acres of forested wetlands in southeastern Virginia and northeastern North Carolina. A single channel stretches through the heart of the swamp, north to south, connecting the rivers near Virginia City with the Albemarle Sound. The waterway was heavily used by peat moss harvesters over a hundred years ago but has now been abandoned to us sightseers. And it is a perfectly beautiful, unspoiled sight to see. The trees are thick cedars hanging heavily with Spanish moss over the canal, whose water is stained black by tannic acid. "Safe enough to drink," the lockmaster told me, though I wouldn't touch the stuff except under the most dire emergency.

A leisurely full-day cruise takes me back to scenes of Bogart and Hepburn aboard the *African Queen*. The water is soundless, but the forest echoes with the calling of birds, bobcats, black bear, tree climbers of various kinds, and countless insects. I didn't have to get out to push, so I can't report on the leeches. "Enchanting" is a bit overused among the crustier Brits, but the word fits perfectly here. Exhilarating, captivating, and, yes, enchanting.

KaRump! I felt *Ka Ching*'s stern give a lurch to the left and heard the sickening, heavy burst of vibration spread up from below. I slapped the throttles to idle and moved the transmissions to neutral. Twenty miles into the swamp, one or even two of my propellers had found a deep stump or submerged log. I checked behind the boat but saw no sign of an object in the black inky water. At least *Ka Ching* was adrift and not aground. I sure would hate to get out of the boat and do a Bogart imitation here.

One of the hazards of making solid contact with a submerged object, besides damage to the propeller, is the potential for the force of the collision to pull the shaft free from the transmission. The shaft and propeller could then drop out of the hole at the bottom of the boat and fall away, leaving the water to flow freely into the bilge and sink the boat. The first check, then, was to open the engine covers to be sure that water was not flowing in from the shaft pits. They seemed OK; no water rushing in on either side. Any damage must be confined to the props and shafts. That done, I remounted the bridge and tentatively put the port transmission into forward. Turning at idle speed, there seemed to be no unusual vibration from a possible bent propeller or bent shaft. It was a different story when I engaged the starboard shaft; a heavy vibration signaled that at least one of the three propeller blades on the starboard side had been curled up like a potato chip.

Gib

And so it was that on the evening of August 5, *Ka Ching* limped on one engine into a boat repair yard in Portsmouth, Virginia. Across the harbor were the ships and cranes of the Portsmouth Naval Shipyard, a major U.S. Navy submarine and surface ship repair facility. *Ka Ching* was lifted out of the water by a large gantry and placed on chocks to allow repair of the starboard propeller and prop shaft. The little boat took its place among many vessels from all parts of the world undergoing refitting in the repair yard. Its neighbors were large sailboats, motor yachts, trawlers, and even a rear-wheel paddle steamer. Some were old battered boats with barnacle-encrusted propellers and rudders. Others were sleek luxury yachts completing expensive refittings. The yard had an air of quiet competence, as if to say, "If you have a problem with your boat, we can fix it."

Gib thought the repairs to the propeller would take only a couple of days. He let his children know that he expected to meet them in New York on the weekend of August 20–22. However, again he hit the snags that had bedeviled his trip; the replacement propeller and other parts took three weeks to arrive. On August 15 Hurricane Charlie blew through Portsmouth with lots of rain and a few puffy breezes; it was far from the killer storm it had been in Florida.

On August 23, while *Ka Ching* was still on chocks in the repair yard at Portsmouth, Gib flew to Miami to see me again for a follow-up in the clinical research trial. Marcia came up from Key West to spend a little time with him and found Gib in a terrible state of hygiene. The sinus surgery at the Mayo Clinic had destroyed his sense of smell, and this was compounded by his inability to take a shower in *Ka Ching* because of the cramped location and his weakened arms. He had also given up using deodorant because he could not smell that anything was amiss. He was wearing pants and a dirty T-shirt that stank to high heaven. She took him out to buy a new set of clothes and got him washed up in time for his visit with me.

When I examined Gib, I found that he could no longer lift his right arm, though the fingers still worked pretty well. He fed himself by propping his right arm on the tabletop to hold the funnel attached to the PEG tube and poured in cans of Jevity Plus that he held in his left hand. Unfortunately his left arm was also beginning to show signs of weakening.

I knew that it was now a race against time. Would he be able to finish the voyage or would the progressive paralysis of his arms force him to give up? I really did not know which was going to win this race. Gib might have had his own misgivings about this, but neither of us shared our fears with the other. He returned to *Ka Ching* with my congratulations and best wishes, and another supply of trial medication. Marcia sent him more boxes of liquid food, this time the higher-calorie Jevity 1.5, which provided him with over 3,200 calories a day.

The following column appeared in the *Citizen* the next week.

REFLECTIONS ON MAGIC, LOSS,
AND SEASONS IN THE SUN
By Gib Peters

"You certainly are keeping a stiff upper lip," Doc Bradley intoned distractedly as he pulled against my straining right bicep. I wondered sarcastically just how my upper lip was connected to the arm muscles he was testing. He moved to the left arm and did the same pull-against-me test with the other bicep. Then he turned to engage me with a clear gaze: "Your articles in the Citizen *are showing a remarkable capacity for positive thought, but why don't you describe what you're really feeling? You know, about your disease!" It wasn't a light, chiding remark but a serious, heartfelt concern that perhaps I was "covering up" in an unhealthy way.*

He dropped my arms and began working on the fingers and wrists. I gave him a nod but didn't try to answer. Not that he would have understood my spit-mumble any better than anyone else. I have to write notes to him, just as I do with others, because of my inability to speak. Nor did I respond after he was finished pushing and pulling on my neck, back, legs, and toes.

I didn't have the answer.

I collected a couple of renewed prescriptions and accepted his wish for good luck, and caught my flight back from Miami to Savannah, where my cats Faith and Hope were waiting. I was only gone one night, but from their greeting you would have thought that I was smuggling catnip aboard. For weeks after returning, the question "Why don't you describe what you're really feeling?" kept bouncing around in my head. Was I trying to hide my innermost feelings from those around me? Were things worse than I was letting on? Was I fearful that to do so would encourage my reader to turn to the crime report for less mush and more action?

Dig and reflect as I might, I couldn't come up with a satisfactory answer to his question—until this morning. Then it struck me that I was indeed describing my deepest and truest feelings about my experiences on board the Ka Ching. My "stiff upper lip" is, I believe, the way I truly feel about my ALS. I am resigned to my affliction and grateful for the time I have left to enjoy the life I have remaining. I am truly quite content.

Let me tell you why.

When I was diagnosed with Lou Gehrig's disease 18 months ago, I fell into a terrible depression, taking my family and friends to new lows with me. As a diversion, my son Mike and son-in-law George took me on a rafting trip down the Colorado River through the Grand Canyon for a week of camping and exploring. It was there that I was reminded of the unimaginable expanse of time during which our Earth has evolved and the millions of forms that life has taken over the last four billion years; and the inescapable fact that everyone—every single life-form that had been created—had died or was about to die. And I was no exception. I thought backward in time even further to the creation of the universe some six billion years ago.

We are told by Stephen Hawking that every atom of the universe was created at that instant of time from pure energy. God's energy, perhaps. After six billion years of lying around in the form of rocks and dirt, and perhaps being borrowed by other life-forms for their lifetime, a few of those atoms suddenly and temporarily clumped together to form Gib Peters. In another moment in galactic time, they will disassemble and return to their perennial state of waiting until new life calls them up for temporary service. It's the way it works. And I thank God for the tiny portion of His energy that He expended to create the atoms that are, for a moment, me.

Having thus been re-introduced to a new appreciation of time and space and my fleeting place within them, I returned home from the Grand Canyon with a resolve to find happiness for the remainder of my life—not only for the purpose of making the most of God's gift to me, but to help those around me to move through the process of grieving for the anticipated loss. No one else could lead me through it. I had to do so.

So how does a dying man find happiness? I am doing it this way: I've taken one part challenge, mixed it with two parts of planning, and stirred. After it steeps in its own natural juices for a while, I turn it into action and don't look back. My plan was designed to fill a couple of voids still left in my life. The first was a single-handed challenge of the sea that I love so much, together with a final test of my creativity in the face of the hundreds of challenges the sea offers; challenges that are even more acute with only a failing body to meet them.

So much for the recipe; how about the baking? How does one actually create happiness with all the reality competing for attention? I chose an old method known by many. I look carefully for that part of a situation that produces a feeling of gratitude.

If the captain of a big trawler decides to overtake me in a channel at ten knots when I'm doing seven, my vessel is going to be slewed badly by the wake he produces. My reaction could be to rage at him from my bridge and say something nasty on channel 16, but that would only serve to feed in me feelings of anger, retribution, resentment, envy, and even guilt. For the rest of the hour or even the remainder of the day, I'd feel discouraged, defensive, and vanquished. Or I could say a silent "thank you" to the captain of the trawler for setting up one of the challenges I came on this voyage to confront. After all, if everything was silky smooth for two thousand miles, one of my purposes for taking the trip would have been frustrated. "Fantastic," I say. "Let's see if I can minimize the roll this time by holding left rudder and double the rpm on my port engine for about five seconds." The rest of my day is now filled with feelings of either achievement or anticipation for the next trawler that will create another stern wave challenge.

How about missing a 4 p.m. lock schedule by two minutes and facing a night tied up until the next morning? Do I feel gratitude for the schedule makers and lock operators? Why not? Without them, I wouldn't have been able to solve the challenge of a safe tie-up in unknown water, listen to good music while I repaired a couple of worn fenders, and finish the book I started yesterday. How can I be angry, disappointed, depressed, or otherwise ill-tempered about all of that?

Am I avoiding the real state of things in my life? No, that would be a mistake. The happiness I feel would be fleeting and the reality would flood in to smother it. So I will deal with the ugliness first. My disease is fatal; I have a couple of years before I'm "locked in" and vulnerable to colds, pneumonia, and death. I ask myself: Am I doing everything that I responsibly should do about my ALS? Have I done everything I can do about leaving my family as comfortable as I can? If the answers to those two questions are "yes," then I can rest assured that I won't be overtaken by guilt while filling my days with gratitude and happiness.

To answer Doc Bradley, when I attempt to raise a twelve-ounce bottle of water to drain it into my stomach tube, I usually don't make it. My right arm is getting too weak to lift the bottle high enough or hold it long enough. The arm is not working and it never will again. I can accept that, but I can't accept the proposition that I should go home and have somebody else pour it into my tube. My family would slide down that slippery slope with me. I have to find a way to get water down so I can continue challenging trawlers' wakes and make it to New York and back.

So I simply use my left arm to lift my right arm to a higher resting place on the window ledge. Propped up high, I then pass the bottle from my left to my right hand, which is still able to grip and turn. Works every time! That's not a cause for defeat, dejection, and pouting. That's a creative victory! I've met a new challenge and created a solution to beat it, so I can live another day. Isn't that what we all do? Meet the day's challenge so we can live on? Able-bodied or not? It's what Man was designed to do and what I must do for me and for my family.

So I give silent thanks to my body for the muscles that are still working, to the guys who built my boat, and the people who filled the bottles with water. They all contributed, knowingly or unknowingly, to the fulfillment of my dream and gave me the means to celebrate a victory. I feel genuinely good about them, truly pleased with myself, and grateful to God for another moment in his sun.

Gib

As the delay in Portsmouth dragged on, Gib became very frustrated and depressed. He came to realize that he could not do the complete circumnavigation of the eastern United States that he had planned. The most that would be possible would be to reach

New York and turn around to return to Key West. Nevertheless, he still had dreams of traveling across the canal systems of Florida to see his old friend, Dutch, in St. Petersburg on the west coast of Florida, before returning to Key West. He sent news of his change of plans to his nautical buddies.

From: Gib Peters
To: All my family and friends
Subject: The Great Loop

Just a quick report. All is well. Winding up repairs to a propeller and a list of other minor items in Portsmouth, VA. I expect to be under way again early next week.

While here I had a chance to e-mail and "talk" with other boaters who have done the Great Loop through the Erie Canal, Great Lakes, and Mississippi. All have been encouraging, but caution against trying to do it so late in the season. The lost three weeks in Savannah and another three weeks here in Norfolk would have cold weather closing in before I got through Chicago. My plan, therefore, is to take a more leisurely cruise into the Chesapeake and Delaware Bays over the next couple of weeks, before a final sprint to New York. I'll then turn around and retrace my route back home to Florida. I am also planning a diversion through Okeechobee to the west coast to see my good friend, Wally Dutcher. He has been a quadriplegic for over forty-eight years.

Love to you all. Write. I miss your e-mails.

Gib

At last on September 1, *Ka Ching*, with her captain and two able-bodied seacats, Faith and Hope, left Portsmouth, Virginia, and motored into Chesapeake Bay. Gib knew that the bay is notorious for its treacherous shoals and dangerous storms. A quarter of the area of the bay is less than six feet in depth, and it is particularly shallow near the eastern and western shores. At the mouth of the bay is an area called the Middle Ground that is particularly infamous for its shifting sandbars.

However, the weather was calm and *Ka Ching*'s passage up Chesapeake Bay was uneventful. By the evening of September 3 the boat was anchored behind the lighthouse thirty miles up the bay at Point Lookout, Maryland. From there Gib sailed up the Potomac River to Gangplank Marina, located in the heart of Washington, D.C., half a mile south of the National Mall. Gib relaxed now that he had decided to abandon the idea of making the Great Loop. He thought that there was plenty of time to get to New York before winter came. What he failed to consider was the worsening of his ALS, which would prove to be the limiting factor in his ability to complete the return voyage to Key West. In the end, he came to regret the week he spent visiting D.C.'s art galleries and museums.

Gangplank Marina is a large and busy tourist stop for boaters, home to several tour boat lines, one of which is Odyssey Cruises. Gib was very interested in this name because he had already begun to think of his voyage on the Intracoastal as being his own personal odyssey. He brought *Ka Ching* into one of the few transient slips in the marina, where most are taken up with permanent houseboats, some of which are so established that they are two stories tall, with sloping shingle roofs and patio gardens. Many of the other slips are occupied by large private yachts, fast motor cruisers, and luxury sailboats. From the flybridge of his little *Ka Ching*, Gib had a view over the dock house roof to the Washington Monument in the distance.

On September 5, while Gib was still in D.C., Hurricane Frances hit the east coast of Florida. As it traveled across the state, it caused problems for his children in Orlando. Gib sent them an e-mail commiserating about the damage they had suffered. They felt they had gotten off lightly in comparison with the poor people in Palm Beach Country, who had suffered severe damage from Hurricane Frances, and the folks in Port Charlotte and Punta Gorda, who had been wiped out by Hurricane Charley. "Survivor's guilt" is a common syndrome in Florida.

Gib put his feet back on the wheel and steered *Ka Ching* away from the dock of Gangplank Marina on the morning of September 11, 2004. Taking things easy, he motored about thirty miles each day, anchored early, and worked on the boat and his e-mails till it was time to turn in. He returned south down the Potomac River to Point Lookout, and then turned north again into Chesapeake Bay. By the evening of September 15, he was anchored in Patuxent River, Maryland. That day, Hurricane Ivan threatened Key West, and Gib sent worried e-mails to Marcia advising her how to protect herself.

On September 16, he tied up at a marina in Annapolis and attempted to repair a leaking exhaust manifold. He no longer had the strength to remove the bolts that held the manifold to the engine. He wrote to Dick Moody: "It pisses me off! I will have to run the engine compartment blowers all the time till I can get it fixed."

The fiftieth reunion of the Class of '54 was to be held at his alma mater, Shorewood High School in Milwaukee on Saturday, September 18, 2004. Gib knew this would be his last reunion, and he wanted to be there, despite the difficulties of travel. So, early Saturday morning he packed his bag, left *Ka Ching* tied up at the Annapolis marina, took a cab to the Baltimore-Washington International airport, and flew to Milwaukee.

He arrived at Shorewood High School late that afternoon. The dining room was already arranged; two long tables lay covered with red folders holding pictures and stories about the Class of '54 and the names of those who were coming to the reunion. As he looked through the folders, memories of his old classmates came flooding back. When members of the Class of '54 walked into the room, they found him with tears streaming down his cheeks.

It took a great deal of courage for Gib to meet his classmates in his current condition. He had lost more than twenty pounds, and his clothes hung off him. He was drooling much of the time and had great difficulty holding his head up. His right arm was almost useless, so he could not shake hands. Nevertheless, the fact that he had traveled so far to spend the evening with his old classmates, many of whom he had not seen for fifty years, was of enormous importance to all. Despite his ripe smell, many hugged him in appreciation for his being there.

Since he could not speak, Gib composed the following piece for his ReadPlease voice synthesizer. He played it from his computer into the microphone, making sure that he used the New York baritone voice and not that of Crystal Sue.

This is a wonderful moment for me, to be able to see all of you one more time and to be able to say a few words to you through my mouthpiece. He can say the words, but he can't convey the emotion that I feel about their meaning. Suffice it to say that I'm thrilled with the cascade of memories that flood my thoughts as I look into your faces. Memories. That's what reunions are for. To regain lost moments, to remember those who have gone before, and to wish one another farewell for what lies ahead. Memories. Treasure them. For one day it will be all that we have. I've come to understand memories as the roses of December. This is my December. Lou Gehrig's disease will take my body soon, but it can't dim the memories of young friendships, wonderful times, and just the plain silliness we all shared together a half century ago. Time is too short tonight to tell you all my memories, and my ability to convey them is too weak. But I would love to exchange a few memories with each of you by e-mail in the months to come. E-mails I can still handle. Thank you, Barbara and Nan and all those who brought us together tonight. And thanks to each of you, my friends, for the countless roses you have given me tonight.

Gib could not stay all evening, because he was having trouble with his PEG tube, the result of poor hygiene. He spent Saturday night in the emergency department of the local hospital in Shorewood, getting a new tube inserted and receiving treatment for a skin infection around the gastrostomy hole. When he flew back to Annapolis and *Ka Ching* the next day, he developed a urinary tract infection and had to get it treated in an emergency department in Annapolis.

From: Gib Peters
To: Marcia Peters
Subject: Bladder infection

I picked up a bladder infection somewhere along the way, which I ignored initially till I could deny it no longer. I was making my way up the west coast of the Chesapeake Bay and had spent the night at anchor between Greenbury Point and the Naval Station at Dungan Bay about two miles northeast of Annapolis. I spent a fitful night and awoke early in a feverish sweat. Time to find a doctor. I motored back across the inlet to Bert Jabin's Yacht Yard, where the lady behind the counter read my note that said: "I need a doctor." She sat me down, called a local hospital, and ordered a cab. Nice people. At the hospital, a nurse asked a half dozen questions, three of which were related to my insurance. She added a note to her report: "Unable to speak."

That's when it became interesting. From that time on, after the doctor came in, the nurse became the sole source of information about me and I was relegated to the status of an incompetent, deaf and dumb bystander. "Is he allergic to any medications?" I shook my head but was ignored. "Does he have pain when he urinates?" I nodded with some emphasis. Ignored again. Hey, what am I? Chopped liver? How in the hell would she know? Ask me! After two more questions to the nurse, I found my clipboard and scribbled a note. "I am competent, I can hear, but I am unable to speak. Ask me!" The young doctor looked at me, apologized, and turned his attention and interrogation to me.

Gib

His urinary infection was resolving with antibiotic solution that he poured into his PEG tube three times a day, when he cast off from Bert Jabin's Yacht Yard on September 21 and continued his cruise up Chesapeake Bay. Though the weather was relatively fair, the waves made his head bobble around uncontrollably as he rode the flybridge eleven feet above the center of rotation of the boat. The transit up the west coast, past Baltimore and the Aberdeen Proving Ground, gave him some warning about his limits and those of *Ka Ching* in handling the tricky conditions on Chesapeake Bay.

~~~~~

Gib received a flood of e-mails from many of the old classmates he had seen at his fiftieth high school reunion. Several said how much he had touched their hearts with his courage in facing ALS. Bruce Larkin, who had been on the diving team at Shorewood High School with Gib, admonished him not to give up hope. Gib replied:

> **From:** Gib Peters
> **To:** Bruce Larkin
> **Subject:** On giving up

On "giving up," Bruce, I don't know what to say. My doctors tell me there is no cure and that the disease moves relentlessly to complete "locked in" and death due to breathing complications, although Doc Bradley reports that ALS sometimes arrests its progress and plateaus. But that's rare. So far, no plateau. I am on the only medication known to delay death but not avoid it. I'm also on an experimental drug, which appears to have no effect that I can see. Still, I do have hope and faith; hope that the disease might arrest, and faith that in another twenty years someone will figure out how to regenerate the dying nerves. Our good friend Wally Dutcher has lived with that hope for almost fifty years. In the meantime I intend to live as though there's no tomorrow. I'm not going to shrivel up in a rocking chair. If you'll forgive a memory from our diving, instead I'm going to my grave with a twenty-four-inch hurdle step to the end of the board, a full-weight press with every ounce of my being, and a toes-together launch toward the ceiling for a full-twisting forward two-and-a-half on the way down to a perfect, no-splash entry, yelling TEN! TEN! TEN!

Gib

~~~~~

At the northern end of Chesapeake Bay is the Chesapeake and Delaware Canal, which connects Chesapeake and Delaware Bays. Gib entered the C&D Canal from the west through the wide inlet from the bay and soon passed under the high bridge at Chesapeake City, Maryland. He did not take time to turn to the south, into the Mooring Basin with its elegantly restored old town. Instead he motored east along the canal under a number of bridges, including two contrasting suspension bridges at St. Georges. To the east is the old bow-shaped bridge and to the west the new suspension bridge that looks like a delicate fan. From St. Georges, the C&D Canal continues to its eastern end near Delaware City, Delaware.

Construction of the C&D Canal first started in 1804 and was not completed until 1829. The canal initially had four locks to raise and lower ships passing from one bay to the other, but in 1927 the high sections were excavated and the C&D Canal became a sea level passage. In some parts, the canal is only a few feet below the level of the surrounding countryside, while in other places, such as St. Georges, the land rises to a height of sixty feet on both sides.

The canal is wide and deep enough to accommodate large seagoing tankers and container ships that dwarfed little *Ka Ching*. Gib wrote that they "sometimes creep up from behind if one's not alert. I often thought seriously about mounting a rearview mirror over my head, but it never went further than 'Yeah, sure!'"

From the C&D Canal, Gib steered *Ka Ching* on a southerly course down Delaware Bay to Cape May, New Jersey, where he turned east into the Cape May Canal. This three-mile-long waterway links the southern end of Delaware Bay with Cape May Harbor. It was constructed as an emergency measure in 1942 to provide shipping with a protected route that avoided going out into the Atlantic Ocean to round Cape May Point, where Nazi U-boats were lurking.

From Cape May Harbor, Gib turned *Ka Ching* northeast into the New Jersey Intracoastal Waterway (ICW) on his way toward New York. Now he was running past one small tourist town after another along the Jersey shore. While development along the beaches is extensive, he saw few tall buildings until he reached Atlantic City, with its high-rises like the Trump Taj Mahal and Casino.

Gib did not find this part of the ICW particularly attractive, and it was with some relief he that he passed Atlantic City on September 27 and continued northward. The protection of the ICW ends at Manasquan Inlet, and from there he had to brave the open Atlantic Ocean for the thirty-mile run into New York Harbor.

But on September 28, Gib's luck ran out; the weather broke. An early fall storm blew in from the Atlantic to affect the whole of the New Jersey–New York seaboard. This forced him into a marina in Barnegat Bay some ten miles south of Manasquan

Inlet, where he was stuck for what seemed like forever.

Gib had promised his children that they would spend a long weekend with him when he arrived in New York. Originally Gib had expected to be there for the weekend of July 4. Now it looked as though it would be early October before he reached the city. Marcia decided to let her children have Gib to themselves for the New York visit, even though October 2 was their thirty-ninth wedding anniversary. The kids had not seen their father for more than four months, while she had seen him each month in Miami on his research visits. Moreover, she was exhausted from the hurricanes, managing the home nursing agency, and keeping Gib supplied with whatever he needed.

Gib was now using his feet not only to steer the boat but also to manage the engine controls. He had become remarkably skillful at steering *Ka Ching* in this way. To the casual observer he looked extremely relaxed as he leaned back in his captain's chair with his feet up. He brought her into the marina at Barnegat Bay on September 28, and was trapped there by the continuing bad weather, almost in sight of New York Harbor. This e-mail became his next column in the *Key West Citizen*.

From: Gib Peters
To: All my family and friends
Subject: New York in sight

If I get up on the bridge this morning and stand on my tip-toes, I can just about see the Statue of Liberty fifty miles to the North. I'm so close to my northernmost goal that I'm tempted to minimize the hazards and mentally shorten the distance between Barnegat Bay and New York harbor to justify starting my engines and casting my lines.

But the lessons that I learned while flying have transferred easily to marine navigation. While teaching flying to private and commercial students, I found that lawyers and doctors were the most dangerous pilot candidates; they are skip-ahead achievers who expected to fly on schedule and damn the weather. As a class, those guys (me included) always wanted to push the limits and sometimes paid the ultimate price for their impatience and overconfidence. I refused to endorse one such hotshot for solo for no other reason than lack of weather judgment. He was technically ready, but not emotionally equipped to be a good pilot. He went off in a huff.

So "I can make it" is no longer in my lexicon. I pulled into a non-transit marina looking for safe harbor late on Tuesday evening, just an hour before gale-force winds and heavy rain hit the New Jersey coast, and I write today from my assigned slip. Yesterday morning the marina manager looked up over the counter to see a sleepless, unshowered, foul-weather-gear-clad sailor offering his best pantomime about the events of the night before. This marina is huge. Until I walked in at 9 a.m., he had no idea that *Ka Ching* was nestled in among 150 other vessels at one of the few open slips. "Looking for safe harbor last night; tied up at 1-10. Can you assign me a slip for a few days before I transit to NY?" I scribbled. "New York!" he said in amazement. "You aren't going to New York any time soon, my friend. That's quite a storm out there. And as for a slip, we have no slips for transients, but I'll fix you up. Take 5-17, just off the clubhouse. Hook up and hunker down."

"Thanks. What do I owe you?" I wrote. "FREE," he wrote on my clipboard. "That's a storm, and I don't have a transient fee schedule or corresponding buttons on the cash register. Impossible to charge you. See? You're my guest for the duration."

Now, I didn't show up on a garbage barge, and I knew damn well he had a way to charge me but clearly didn't want to. He and I both knew that any encouragement to sit it out would be a smart sailor's move. He was doing his part to add to my supply of caution. He didn't have to, but he's a sailor. Another one of a hundred really fine people I've met and dealt with since leaving Key West. I'm continually impressed with the sensitivity and charity of those I touch.

I wonder about how my affliction and handicaps influence those I encounter. They are certainly aware of them. When I make my way down the docks or snoop around the marinas and nearby shops, I hold my head up with my left hand under my chin like Auguste Rodin's "The Thinker." The pose sometimes covers up my inability to hold my head up naturally, but up close the dribbling and drooling give me away every time. My lips are all but paralyzed and offer little control over the flow of saliva. Distressing as hell. Offers to lift a bag of laundry, a case of bottled water, or to help plug into a 30-amp shore power circuit come out of nowhere. People are quick to pick up my weaknesses and cover-ups, despite my best efforts to finesse them. And just as quick to help.

Charity, did Doc Bradley say? Sure. It's built in to us all. Whether hardwired into the genes or learned early in our formative years, the urge to "give a hand" seems to pop out on impulse all around. I had never given even a wisp of a thought to being the trigger for that reflexive attention or the focus of the action that follows. I've always been on the other side; the reactor and the helper. Being the recipient is an ambivalent place that's both uncomfortable and comforting. I don't like it. But like it or not, it's my time. I'm becoming weaker and more dependent.

I promised a look into the petri dish when I arrived at the halfway mark of my venture to see how the organism that is me has changed since leaving Key West back in May. It has changed. My mind is stronger, clearer, more focused and aware than when I left. My sensitivity to the world that passes my bow is on full gain with no abatement of the highs and lows of new experiences. My world around me rings with truth and order and beauty. Yes, the sky is bluer. The shrillness of pain flares occasionally, but the quiet sub-base beat of a distant mother's heart is ever-present. Spiritually, I'm growing too. E-mail dialog with my friends and relatives, reflection, and reading have sharpened my thinking and have turned me in directions that are ever more satisfying. My emotional connection to life is strong and growing stronger as my body becomes weaker.

My arms are at my sides more, although the ALS has been slower to weaken the finger muscles. This still allows me to toss my arms into position for my fingers to do their work. Occasionally I must give up the effort to turn a wrench or crimp some heavy wires. My back and neck are measurably weaker. However, I've found that tilting the captain's chair back at just the correct angle allows me to balance my head right at the top of its center of gravity without straining the neck muscles fore and aft or side to side. I'm sure I look like a life-size bobble-head doll at the helm in choppy water, but in this position I end the day without ache or pain. My legs are OK; not strong, but adequate. Muscle shrinkage has left them weaker, but I don't think the nerves controlling them are dying yet. Breathing is good; the last test showed my lungs to be unaffected thus far and still functioning at 120 percent of normal. (Due to hyperventilated free diving when in the Navy, I'm told. Go Navy.)

The sum of all of that progress and regression has produced a very alive and alert organism that creeps around veeeery carefully on *Ka Ching*. My vessel offers plenty of handholds and tries to keep her deck under me regardless of the weather, although there are limits. My highest-risk activity now is moving from the foredeck to the afterdeck along the narrow walkways next to the cabin. If the pitching motion is too severe, I just don't go; or if it's absolutely necessary, then I wear a life jacket. However, even if I fell overboard, I'm not 100 percent confident that I could get back in. I've rigged a rope ladder up to the platform with some handholds for such an emergency. I plan to have reinstalled the dive ladder that was taken off when the dinghy was mounted. That should provide a second method of reboarding.

My slow, awkward, and carefully studied movements today remind me of a younger time when I commuted Central Expressway from Plano to Dallas each day. After a grueling day I was motoring home, anxious to squeeze my bride and my kids. I lined up behind a slow-moving Cadillac to wait my turn at the change-only toll booth and crept toward the basket, now tantalizingly close ahead in front of the Cadillac.

"Yea, yea, go, go!" I coached the driver ahead. The Cadillac slowly eased into position next to the yawning change basket. The window slowly slid down to full open, and the silver-headed driver's attention turned to select the coins from what must have been a car treasury in the center console.

"Hey, that's Mr. Thompson. I didn't know he was still out and about," I thought to myself. A long twenty seconds went by as he selected three quarters and slowly turned toward the open window. Mr. Thompson was founding partner of Thompson and Knight, a large and prestigious law firm in Dallas that represented the likes of Texas Instruments, E-Systems, and J.C. Penney. Mr. Knight was a large benefactor of my nonprofit, TAGER (The Association for Graduate Education and Research). "OK, Mr. Thompson, my castle awaits; just toss in those coins and give her the gas!" The traffic flowed past on the right and left as Mr. Thompson raised his left arm carefully up and through the window toward the basket. Clink. One quarter. One! What's the matter, Thompson, old boy, three quarters too heavy?

The seconds drifted by as he returned his attention to the treasury. After a long moment the left hand re-extended toward the basket. Clink. Two down. "Way to go, Tommy! Let's fire in that last one and lay some rubber! My margarita awaits!" Mr. Thompson's treasury must have run out of quarters just then, because I could distinctly see him counting out the last twenty-five cents in smaller change. "COME ON!" I screamed at the windshield. He didn't hear me, of course, but it made me feel better. The hand extended once more toward the basket; clink, clink, ping! One coin, a dime or a nickel, struck the lip of the basket and bounced out onto the pavement. "To hell with it, Tommy. Blow through it; I'll take care of it when I get up there!" He didn't hear that either.

The big heavy door of the Cadillac opened slightly and rested against the basket with just enough room for a left foot to emerge and find its way to the pavement. It shuffled its way toward the back of the door to allow the right foot to follow and provide a sure place for the old body to bring itself erect and emerge from the car. "Oh my God, he's going after the damn nickel!"

In dramatic exasperation, I put my arms around the steering wheel, shut my eyes tightly, and let my head drop forward to the wheel. BEEP! "Oh, noooo." I had blown my horn at the old fart. "I'm dead. I am such a self-centered shit. What is wrong with you, Peters? Get your ass out there and help the man!" But I didn't. My embarrassment overwhelmed the charity that was hardwired into my bones. It was suppressed, trammeled, and forgotten. I spent the next minutes avoiding any backward glance he might make. But he never noticed me or my impatient and self-indulgent profile while recovering his nickel, and dropped it into the basket. I was devastated when I finally pulled away from that toll gate. I still am.

Wherever you are, Mr. Thompson, please forgive me. I didn't understand.

Gib

~~~~~

The bad weather around New York continued for several more days, and Gib wisely waited out the storm. On Friday, October 1, blue skies appeared, and he judged it safe to head for New York Harbor.

Though Gib was fifty miles from the Statue of Liberty as the crow flies, he still had to motor up the last part of the Jersey ICW to the Manasquan Inlet, which lay thirty miles north of Barnegat Bay, running inside a long strip of outer barrier islands that separates the ICW from the Atlantic Ocean. Then he had to steer *Ka Ching* out into the open Atlantic Ocean for thirty miles before rounding Sandy Hook peninsula, which forms the southern lip of the entrance to New York Harbor. And then he had another sixteen miles to go before reaching the Lower Bay and the Statue of Liberty.

Bright and early on October 2, Gib steered *Ka Ching* out of the Manasquan Inlet, through the narrow passage between the breakwater to the north and the beach off Ocean Avenue to the south, and past a few early morning fishermen hopefully casting their lines. Despite the recent storms, the Atlantic was as calm as a millpond.

Late that evening he found an anchorage just inside New York Harbor to the west of Sandy Hook lighthouse. Built in 1764, it is the oldest working lighthouse in the United States. He anchored to the south of the Coast Guard station and the dock for the high-speed catamaran ferry from Manhattan. From his anchorage he looked eastward to the mostly derelict buildings of Fort Hancock, built as an Army barracks in 1899 and used to house and train troops during World Wars I and II. This National Historic Landmark is now run by the National Park Service; though many of the barrack buildings are boarded up, some are used for summer teaching and research programs.

Gib cruised into New York Harbor on October 3. He was soon stopped by a Coast Guard launch, owing to security measures put into place followed the 9/11 attack on the World Trade Center. They had never seen anyone steer a boat with his feet before. Gib reassured them that he was not a terrorist, and the Coast Guard released him. He toured New York Harbor and the East and Hudson Rivers. He wanted to get a good view of the skyscrapers of Manhattan. He drew many curious stares from passengers on the harbor ferries.

Late that afternoon he tied up at a marina at Great Kills Harbor on Staten Island. The name Great Kills derives from the Dutch word *kill*, meaning a channel or creek. It comes from the time when what is now Manhattan was known as New Amsterdam and was a Dutch colony.

Gib moved to a little anchorage on the northwest side of Liberty Island on October 4, from where he looked past the back of the Statue of Liberty to the fabulous views of downtown Manhattan while getting the boat cleaned up for his children's visit and working on his e-mails. On Thursday, October 7, he moved from Liberty Island, past the tour boats and Ellis Island, to Liberty Harbor Marina on the New Jersey side of New York harbor. This is just across the Hudson River from Manhattan and provided easy access when his family arrived.

Gib and Marcia loved New York and would often go to two Broadway shows in one day when they visited. They had taken their young children on a number of visits to the city, and Gib wanted to reintroduce them to its spectacular sights and sounds. Gib particularly loved the show *The Producers*, and a week before arriving in New York he had ordered online six matinee tickets.

While waiting for his children to arrive in New York, he mused on the continuity of life from one generation to another.

His thought-provoking message went out to everyone on his list server and was later published in the *Key West Citizen*.

From: Gib Peters
To: All my family and friends
Subject: Remembrance of things past

As a child—well, an infant, really—my mother would find moments of peace by laying me on the carpet and dropping a piece of string onto the floor next to me. She had discovered that an old butcher cord was my all-time favorite toy. You might scoff at the likelihood of my remembering such a thing, but I do; as clearly as any memory I have, as vividly as anything that makes a profound impression on one's mind during a lifetime. Having two ends, the string had the capacity to "follow" itself wherever I pulled it. When I tugged at one end, the other would trail behind and be affected in exactly the same way along its length. I was absolutely absorbed by its motion and would spend long minutes among the forest of potted plants, towering end tables, and flat carpeted plains trying to sort out the mystery of the phenomenon. My mother confirmed my memory of it years later. Had I the vocabulary, I would have called the concept "communication." Making a change in something distant by affecting something near.

My infant fascination with string extended later to tin-can "telephones" to my playmate's house across the alley, sending "messages" up my kite string to a buddy standing in a field beyond, battery-operated Morse code clickers wired into every room, ham radio as a teen, and eventually into the Navy as a radio operator.

Why did I study law years later? Because I couldn't handle the math required for my yearning to be an engineer—a prerequisite,

I thought, of being a communications system maker. But I soon discovered that words substituted nicely for numbers and opened broad avenues for communication that didn't exist on the slide rule. But law was a false start for me too. Although admitted to the bar, I never practiced law. I just used it in my career to serve my need to "make a change in something distant by affecting something near." I discovered, too, that I didn't fit into a driven, Type A personality mold, determined to command men and claw to the top. In my heart of hearts, I was really a teacher, a counselor, and an advisor. "Personality" appraisals throughout my career all pointed to the same conclusion, even though I tried to skew the results to come out as the "commander" type that was my image of success. College administrator, business law teacher, flight instructor, financial advisor, and occasional writer validated those tests. In the end, they were happy careers.

Those are all behind me now, except for writing, as you can see. As the usual means of communication close behind me, the word processor is now my "string" to the outside world. My speech is nonexistent, signing is a foreign language, and my pantomime is silly. But if I tug at one end of the keyboard, I've found that the reader at the display end is sometimes affected. I'm still complete.

I'll lose the ability to move my fingers over the keyboard in a year or so. But I've tested a Morse code key connected to my laptop to create letters, sentences, and ideas. I'll use whatever part of my body that is still able to move to operate the switch while it's my good fortune to remain alive. Yes, I still remember Morse code. So I still expect to be able to pull the string and be able to teach for a little while longer. I like that.

"Then, Professor, what do you profess? Whom do you teach?" My response to the first is one man's philosophy of life and death, his place in the world and his notion of legacy. My response to the second is my contemporaries, as long as they welcome my professions.

But I've recently become absorbed with the idea of reaching back to the past for instruction from my progenitors, and to leave some thoughts to my heirs and descendants. Unlike communicating with contemporaries, such "vertical" communication from predecessor to descendant is necessarily a one-way transmission. We can't talk to past generations, but we have a capacity to influence those who follow us. We leave "stuff" to our kids; why not impressions, descriptions, and ideas? I'll omit from this list "instructions" and "advice." These are to be found in the pedantic, sanctimonious writings called legacy wills, which are created solely for that purpose.

My prayer is that my children's children will have the framework solidly in place to make their own good decisions and to chart their own true courses. They will do so anyway and won't need my advice. But perhaps, just perhaps, they will look back in time to the notes of an ancestor named Gib Peters, about how he lived and died. Perhaps they will see a bit of themselves and understand more clearly the deep-seated drives that stir them to pull a string, fly a plane, avoid math, teach another, or search for God.

My memory of my ancestors is frustratingly shallow. I recall my grandmother's dark, wallpapered rooms over a noisy bar in Antigo, Wisconsin. A few colorless scatter rugs covered holes in well-worn linoleum over boards that creaked when you walked over certain places. In the winter, it was cold in every room except the kitchen, which was over-warmed by a wood stove that grandma used for cooking. Potatoes and bread. And perhaps meat when someone killed a deer. Her second husband was a benign alcoholic who dribbled chewing tobacco on his shirt and smelled of the smoky musk of the bar downstairs and the woods where he cut trees. I have an impression that my grandmother was not a happy woman. I never learned about her girlhood, her joys and heartaches, her struggles to survive, or how she died. Nor do I recall anything about her parents or those who came before.

How nice it would be to have an old letter with a few lines from the French-Canadian trapper who married an Indian girl in a trading post on the shores of Lake Michigan, called Miliokee, which became Milwaukee. My dad mentioned this vague bit of oral family history just once. But he had nothing more to offer me about his predecessors. So I am writing these musings mainly for my grandchildren, great-grandchildren, and those who follow, to tell them who I was and what I did. It makes me feel like I'm connecting and that my life will be remembered and noted favorably across a few generations.

And so I write.

But words are one thing. To touch an artifact from the writer is another. I hope to leave a few personal time capsules for my descendants on my return trip to Key West. Before leaving, I raided the dark depths of my top dresser drawer, where I kept a small box of cast-off smooth-worn jewelry, old but still-working Timex watches, campaign buttons, club pins, and foreign coins, to name but a few. During my boat trip up the East Coast, I took note of a number of suitable places where I might drop anchor, launch the dinghy, and carry bureau-drawer treasure ashore for burial. I'll revisit those places on my return trip and carry back home a carefully drawn map of the spot I selected. I will leave to my descendants a challenge: Find your way to the "treasure," dig up the old guy's idea of a personal time capsule, and see if the artifact makes any connection.

They might find a Shorewood High School class ring of 1954 in a glass bottle, a University of Wisconsin Hoofers ski pin with a

Rose Bowl button sealed in a plastic Ensure container, or a pocketful of long-forgotten coins from Old Europe in a triple-plastic-wrapped, soldered tin can. Or a hundred other nominal value artifacts from a distant personal past.

They will be welcome to take what they find, replace it with something of their own, and rebury it to whet their own children's sense of discovery and connection. I like the idea. I feel as though I am connecting, teaching, communicating, and loving across the barriers of time. I think I've figured out how to pull the string. I'd love to be able to see if the other end moves.

Gib

Mike, Lisa, Kim, George, and Lynnea arrived in New York on the evening of Thursday, October 7. They had originally planned that Gib would stay in the hotel with them, but he found it easier to sleep on his boat. They arranged to meet at 10:00 a.m. Friday in Grand Central Station by the information booth under the big brass clock. Gib traveled from Liberty Harbor Marina to Manhattan by the Port Authority Trans Hudson Subway, known to all as the PATH, and was waiting for them when they arrived.

His children immediately perceived that Gib was having problems with hygiene. Their first impression was of the smell of fish, seawater, and diesel fuel, intimately mixed. Of course, Gib could not smell this delightful concoction. They were shocked to see how much weight he had lost. Despite twelve cans a day of liquid food, he had not been able to keep up with the calorie requirements of the physical activity needed to run *Ka Ching*. Mike, who had not seen his dad for six months, thought, "Wow! He is so thin! So frail! How in the world did he make it this far?" George was also taken aback. He thought, "How has he possibly managed to get the boat to New York by himself? And more important, how is he going to take it all the way back to Key West?"

Gib's kids took him back to their hotel and got him cleaned up. They then took him to the top of the Empire State Building, where he reintroduced them to the sights of Manhattan. When they came out of the elevator at the ground floor of the building, they realized that Gib was exhausted and suggested that he return to *Ka Ching* and rest up for tomorrow's excursions. Gib insisted on making his own way back to the Liberty Harbor Marina by the PATH, so they dropped him off at the nearest subway station, went back to the hotel bar, and spent a couple of hours reminiscing. They talked about their life with Gib and the effect that the ALS was having on the whole family.

Unfortunately Gib took the wrong branch of the PATH and found himself traveling north toward Hoboken. A kind fellow-traveler redirected him, and the next morning Gib sent him an e-mail to express the gratitude he had been unable to convey at the time since he couldn't speak.

The next morning, Saturday, October 9, bright and early, the five of them went to visit Gib on *Ka Ching*. They took a water taxi from Battery Park across the Hudson to Liberty Harbor. The temperature was hovering around the freezing point. Despite the cold, Gib was full of smiles and happy mumblings to see his children. The boat's cabin was not a pretty sight and had quite an odor to it. They remembered what Gib and *Ka Ching* looked like in the years before ALS and the voyage up the Intracoastal Waterway; Mother Nature had taken a toll on both of them. They embraced, and nobody held back their tears.

Gib wanted to have lunch at Sardi's Restaurant on Broadway, where the theater stars hang out, so they all took the PATH back to Manhattan. At Sardi's, though Gib wasn't able to eat, the fact that his children enjoyed the food made him very happy. They sat around a big table, and Gib gazed about with a smile that wouldn't go away. They were cracking the usual Peters family jokes, ripping each other to shreds, and he couldn't get enough of it. They could hear Gib's mumbled laughs followed by some coughs, but Gib had no speech to be able to take part in the repartee. Afterward, they said that it was the quietest they had seen him in his whole life, but also the happiest.

In an e-mail a few days later, Gib told Mike, "I was the proudest dad ever to walk down Broadway. And when guys looked at me with three gorgeous women on my arm and two bodyguards trailing, I just thought: 'Eat your hearts out, fellas!'"

That afternoon they went to the matinee of *The Producers*. The seats were upstairs in the loge section with a perfect view of the stage. They were all emotionally drained by the visit, and before the curtain went up Gib took a quick catnap. Once the show started, however, he didn't take his eyes off the stage for a moment. While a wonderful time was had by all, George watched his father-in-law during the show and couldn't help wondering, "What are his thoughts? How much longer do we have with him? Will this be the last time we all spend quality time together?"

Early on Sunday, October 10, 2004, Gib set off from New York to make his way back to Key West. He had hoped to do the Great Loop, but that was not to be. Even reaching Key West was going to be a stretch. He was not the same man who had left his Riviera Canal dock twenty weeks before. He had lost a lot of weight and most of the use of his arms, particularly the right one. He probably had only 5 percent of the normal number of motor neurons in the bulbar region of his brain, while the number in his cervical spinal cord was probably just 20 percent of normal. The respiratory muscles in his chest wall and diaphragm had less than 50 percent of their normal nerve supply, and even his leg muscles were beginning to be affected.

Because of the terrible toll wrought by ALS, Gib now had to retrace the route back to Key West with much less physical strength—and in deteriorating weather. He knew that he must speed up if he was to have any hope of completing his odyssey. Whenever possible, he pushed *Ka Ching* to ten knots. He traveled for longer stretches each day, which exhausted him and left little time to communicate with family and friends. The e-mails and articles took him longer to write since his right hand continued to weaken. In the end, he was typing with just his left index finger.

Gib retraced the thirty-mile dash through the open Atlantic and then ducked into the Manasquan Inlet at 3:00 p.m. that Sunday. He was grateful to be finished with the open ocean and thought that the worst of the journey was now behind him. Little did he know what awaited him in the relative safety of the ICW.

He anchored in Barnegat Bay at 6 p.m. and that night wrote about his departure from New York Harbor and the memories it revived.

From: Gib Peters
To: All my family and friends
Subject: On the homeward leg

A cold front moved through New York during the night, bringing with it a new urge to be under way again, but this time south to Florida and home. The trip from Key West to New York stretched five months into the late fall season, partly because of the generator delays but also because I felt that I should "spare" *Ka Ching*'s engines from the added stress that higher speeds would bring. I felt that if the engines were babied during the leg north, I had a better chance of making the 2,000 miles to New York than if I had pushed them at higher speeds. There was one other reason that the trip north was so long: I was frankly just dawdling, enjoying the sunsets, the sights along the Intracoastal Waterway, and the time to rest, think, and write.

I started the engines, tested the transmissions by shifting each briefly to forward and reverse and watching for a slight movement while still at the dock. *Ka Ching* tugged nervously against her lines, telling me that she was ready to go. Hope and Faith were safely curled up with one another on the rocking chair, the fairway looked clear of other vessels, so I pulled in the last line holding me to the dock and mounted the bridge. I certainly don't mean to attract attention while maneuvering, but inevitably I do so. My arms and hands are no longer useful, so they remain at my sides while seated at the helm as my legs and feet finesse the helm and transmissions. Other captains and dockhands are fully convinced that I'm showing off a new, lazy man's approach to seamanship. Of course they are exactly right, disabled or not!

I was pleased that I achieved my "short goal," which was to reach New York and have a "Broadway night out" with my kids. My "long goal" had been to return to Key West through the Great Lakes and the Mississippi. But mechanical problems on the way up from Key West had squandered the time that I needed to make the Mississippi route feasible. Now cold fronts moving down from Canada were already sweeping across the Midwest and over the East Coast. The "short goal" of New York and back was it; and to tell the truth, that was probably enough.

I eased my way past a half-dozen finger piers, dodged a Staten Island Ferry being captained by a New York cab driver who just got his captain's license, and offered an affectionate smile to the Lady of the Harbor. Once the turn around the Statue of Liberty was completed and the compass settled onto a southerly heading through New York Harbor, I leaned back in the captain's chair with engines turning at an easy 1,800 rpm, thinking about what lay ahead.

Beyond the Verrazano Bridge and the Swash Channel was the Atlantic Ocean. The twenty-five-plus-mile run south from Sandy Hook to the Manasquan Inlet along the Jersey shore is the only portion of the entire four-thousand-mile trip that has no inland channel but requires travel in open ocean. So it was not without a small amount of exhilaration that I pointed *Ka Ching*'s nose easterly between Coney Island and Sandy Hook for the open Atlantic Ocean. The weather was cold and clear, and the sea calm. There

was a long thirty-second swell coming from some far-away distur-
bance in mid-ocean, but it was a welcome change from the chop-
chop of inland water. After about a ten-mile leg eastward, I eased
the helm southward and set a direct course to the Manasquan
Inlet about three hours distant.

The drone of *Ka Ching*'s engines and the rolling swell soon had
me dreaming about other days and other horizons, and about life
and death. It was probably thirteen years ago, but the memory
is clear. I was fishing in my little seventeen-foot Mako motorboat about ten miles northwest of Key West in forty feet of gin-
clear water. The condition of the water was probably the reason
I wasn't having any luck. But in any case, I was ready to call it a
day, even though it was early afternoon and sunset wasn't until
9 p.m. I started the outboard and headed south toward the
No. 1 day marker of the Calda Channel that would take me back
to Key West Harbor.

On the horizon about three miles ahead and to the left, I
caught a glimpse of another small boat dead in the water and a
figure standing near its center waving both arms—at least, that's
what I imagined it was at three miles. I changed my heading
directly toward the spot and after another minute confirmed that
it was indeed a person waving both arms high over his head and
down to his sides to attract attention. The rule among sailors the
world over is to respond in any way you can to a call for assistance. It is a rule neither I nor anyone I knew ever broke. I turned
up the rpm to maximum and bore down on the figure now about
two miles distant. As I got to within a mile, I noticed that the
water was becoming quite shallow; five feet, four feet, three feet
. . . but there were some six-foot-deep finger channels winding
their way closer to the waving figure. I began running a serpentine
track through these channels.

At a half mile I also began to see several strange, round black humps, about half the size of my small boat, in the water clustered near the other boat, but couldn't make out what they were from this distance. My curiosity was thoroughly aroused by now, and from two hundred yards away the picture became clear. A woman angler had spotted a pod of beached pygmy whales, alive but obviously dying. "Do you have a radio?" she shouted. "Yes. What's up?" I yelled. "Just came upon this pod ten minutes ago. They need help. I can't do much alone." I ran my boat up onto a shoal and got out into knee-deep water to check for life and make a count of the twelve-hundred-pound bodies lying on their sides around me. "Looks like eight to me, and all are still alive, right?" I asked. "I counted ten. I think there are two in the channel behind you," she said.

The water depth where most of them lay was no more than two feet, which left half their bodies exposed above the surface and their blowholes right at surface level, sucking a lungful of air four or five times a minute. The weather was mostly sunny with a mild southeast breeze, so there should be lots of anglers, snorkelers, divers, runabouts, and charters scattered throughout the one hundred square miles around us. We certainly needed every one of them now.

I made my way back to my boat, stepped over the side onto the deck, and reached for my chart and the mike on the VHF radio. The channel selector was already on 16, which is the international calling and distress channel, monitored by most if not all boaters when not actually using another channel. The lady angler in the other boat was now moving from body to body, splashing water on each one to keep the exposed skin from drying out. "Pan pan, pan pan, pan pan. This is motor vessel *Off the Wall* calling on 16 with urgent traffic for whale-watch volunteers. Any station having the ability to assist a stranded pod in the Key West area, shift and listen to channel 78. Out."

Not eleven months before, I had read a long article in the *Key West Citizen* that detailed attempts to rescue another pod that had beached itself somewhere nearby, explaining the theories about this perplexing and sad behavior. A single whale strongly suggested a heart ailment due to lack of some vitamin. But multiple strandings raised other possibilities. No one really knew if it was self-destructive, accidental, fear-driven, disease-driven, or even the full moon, but everyone had an opinion. The article also reported how a large number of people had improvised with the items they had at hand to make the animals more comfortable. A hazy recollection of the details began to take shape as I surveyed the grim scene again.

I shifted my radio to 78, spread the chart in front of me, and verified my location by eyeballing a nearby day marker and a charted but unmarked channel. "Pan pan, pan pan, all stations, this is motor vessel *Off the Wall* calling for volunteers to assist at a multiple whale grounding north of Key West. Stand by to copy position. Break." I let go of the mike button for ten seconds, long enough to make sure the channel was clear and to give any listeners the chance to dig out a pencil. I heard nothing—not even a hint that anybody at all was listening. But I knew that there were a thousand ears straining now to hear the location, whether they could help or not. "All stations, a multiple whale grounding is located approximately one mile east of the No. 1 marker on the Calda Channel at the north end of the Bluefish Channel. There are ten animals lying in two to three feet of water; all appear to be living at this time. Position again is . . ." I repeated the message and asked any station ashore with a phone to call any volunteer agency with an interest in this sort of thing with the location.

I didn't ask for acknowledgment and dropped the mike over the helm wondering what I had on board that would be useful. I turned up an old tube of sunscreen, a beach towel, and a package of soggy donuts. The first two seemed to be the most valuable at the moment, so I slogged my way twenty feet through the shallow water to the first large black body. While making the short trip, I looked up at the horizons to the north and west and saw a dozen or more white bow waves a couple of miles distant moving toward me at high speed, with what appeared to be another six or eight boats coming up Calda Channel in a conga line at thirty knots or more. We were about to have lots of company and, I hoped, lots of blankets and zinc oxide.

My first patient was on her side with a pectoral fin and a large part of her body exposed to the air and sun. I moved around to her large bulbous head, which was on its side but with her mouth down in the water just far enough that her blowhole at the top of her head was slightly above the water level. Her large round right eye was fully open and nervously alert to my movements as I approached and stroked her broad forehead. She didn't react, except that her straining eye was searching for my extended arm and hand hovering over her head. She let out a small, nervous exhalation and quickly took in a fresh breath to hold for another fifteen seconds. I reached down to soak the big towel in the water at my feet and drew it up and over her head and so much of her body as I could without covering the eye or blowhole. It is hard to tell on her dark skin, but she appeared to be getting the first signs of sunburn. I emptied the remaining sun block on her lower half and flukes, rubbing it gently into the gray, dry hide. I didn't bother to read the label to see whether it was waterproof, but then splashed her liberally from end to end anyway. I was sure she was over-heating, but there was no more I could do for her at the moment.

By this time four small boats had pulled into a beached line alongside my own, and a young couple was running through the shallow water in my direction. "What do we do?" I answered with a shrug, "I don't know much about this, but I think they need to be kept cool until somebody who does know gets here." They turned around and shouted something to the other new arrivals who were already splashing toward their own selected beached whale. Another dozen boats had arrived within eight or ten minutes, including a Coast Guard inflatable whose personnel had little more to offer in the way of advice, but did miraculously produce six dark blankets from somewhere on their vessel. They were soon soaked with seawater and covering half a dozen more whale bodies.

One team of eight burly guys managed to get a blanket under one whale which was close to the Bluefish Channel and moved it an inch at a time, with a shouted sailor's cadence of "Now, now, now." They succeeded in getting it into deeper water, but to their palpable disappointment the whale wouldn't leave the shallow water's edge or its pod. They took encouragement, however, from what appeared to be easier breathing with its tremendous weight distributed more evenly and naturally in the water. The crowd had grown to around forty or fifty by 3:00 p.m., including two new arrivals from a whale rescue team and a dolphin research organization, both attempting to take command of the chaos around them.

Exhausted from splashing, lifting, and pushing limp, uncomprehending animals, but assured that they were getting the best first aid available, I staggered back to my Mako. On my way I passed a whale that was lying in the shallowest water farthest from open channel. Sitting in the sand at its head, with legs and knees propped under and against its bulging body, was the lady angler who initially waved me over to the scene. She was alone with the animal, doing her best to hold the blowhole above the water while rocking the huge head imperceptibly to her quiet sobs. But her whale was no longer breathing.

The spell broken, I checked the GPS map to see that New York was now twenty-six miles behind. *Ka Ching*'s engines hadn't missed a stroke over the last two hours, and the open seas remained calm. Manasquan Inlet lay ahead fourteen miles, just over the horizon but not yet in sight. I became captivated by the featureless, infinite line between everything and nothing once again.

What would drive all those animals to choose suicide? Suicide: the act of deliberately killing oneself. But there's the rub. Do animals "choose" an act that will certainly end their lives from among all other acts? It would seem so in the case of those whales. Or were they simply acting from millions of years of "instinct" to seek death when fatally ill?

Will I actively seek death at some point? Dr. Bradley suggested that I would probably consider suicide when the quality of my life degraded to such a level that death seemed the better alternative. He added that he would counsel me at that point, suggesting that I had several options, which he would explain at that time. When he told me of this unhappy option, I was still early in the disease cycle—impaired speech, one weak arm, but otherwise healthy. I was startled by his matter-of-fact offering; it was the clearest message yet that my disease was fatal and untreatable. A year and a half later, I am now entirely speechless, both arms are virtually paralyzed, and my diaphragm is becoming "lazy." And recently for the first time, while in the grip of a simple cold virus, I thought that death would be the better alternative. Breathing through swollen upper respiratory tissues with an ALS-weakened diaphragm was a desperate act of survival for four days and four nights. But the cold ran its course, and I'm back breathing normally again.

Gib

~~~~~~

On Monday, October 11, Gib anchored just north of the Atlantic City inlet, and the following morning motored the short distance across the inlet to Kammerman's Marina, a small dock that provides fuel to the recreational boater. He tied up, refueled, and set off south at a good clip. He was making up for lost time.

Forty miles on, south of Atlantic City, he noticed that Faith and Hope were not aboard.

From: Captain, Motor Vessel *Ka Ching*
To: Dock Master, Atlantic City Marina
Subject: AWOL crew

I stopped to refuel my twenty-nine-foot Sportsbridge at your dock this morning and then continued south on the ICW. After anchoring this afternoon near Cape May, about forty miles from your facility, I discovered that two crewmember cats were not on board. There is a possibility that they jumped ship at your dock and may still be carousing around the fuel pumps or nearby vessels, looking for trouble. Would you please have your dockhands look around to see if you can find them and if you do, please charge them with being AWOL and put them in any handy brig? I will see at that time whether it will be practical to retrieve them.

There are usually a few stray mousers around any marina property, so it's important that I describe them carefully to be sure the real perpetrators are caught. One is male, the other female, and their uniforms are virtually identical. They are black with caramel-colored tiger stripes, with white bibs and bellies and white socks on all fours. Their names are Hope and Faith. They will cunningly ignore their names if called—first, because they probably won't want to be identified; second, because they don't know their names; and third, because they have never before been called by their names. They may, however, respond to certain spit-mumble noises, but that's another story.

They will both have a noticeable salty sailor's gait because they have not been off the boat since they were six weeks old. They are now seven months old. You will notice them to be ill-disciplined, ignoring any order given. Although non-sleeping hours are occupied by personal hygiene and grooming, the few crew duties assigned are performed with careless indifference. When under way, the male will insist on taking the helm watch, at his own pleasure and on his own schedule, by leaping into the captain's lap, assuming a slovenly sailor's posture, and overseeing the helm and compass. From this position he is able to carefully study wind direction and velocity by watching the Conch Republic flag on the bow staff, but will pointedly refrain from warning the captain of changes. He has frequently been put on report for sleeping while on watch, but no amount of spit-mumble lecturing seems to bring a change in behavior.

The female ignores any regular watch duty, but will be alert to any vessel or object on the horizon and warn the captain of any perceived threat from same. Jumping fish and breaching dolphins under the bow will bring her to full battle station status. At other times she will assiduously avoid deck work and small vessel tasks during her tours about the decks, preferring instead to find a sunny place on the afterdeck, rolling onto her back and falling asleep with all fours straight up. Stern warnings about being underfoot have been ineffective.

This background is offered for the purpose of helping you distinguish between these two renegades and others who may be lurking about your docks.

These two AWOL derelicts are not considered dangerous. However, they can be cunning and irritating as hell. Precautions should be taken. The best time of day for a no-risk capture would be during the period of El Gato Siesta: 9 a.m. to 4 p.m. During these hours, they will tend to be lethargic and approachable. However, morning hours prior to 9 a.m. should be avoided as this is a period of high activity and irrational, disrespectful behavior. An example might be instructive for your dockhands. Just prior to daybreak, when the captain is in his vee-bunk enjoying a deep, restful sleep, the two subjects will conspire to make it necessary for the captain to awaken, leave his warm bunk, and open the crew's mess for their breakfast: hardtack and preserved fish mush.

Their methods for disturbing the captain's rest progress from the imaginative and calculating to the cruel. Each will begin the indignity by leaping onto the captain's bunk, sitting at the edge while purring loudly and incessantly for a few minutes, to see if any movement of the captain occurs as a result. If not, they stomp heavily around the captain's prone body to determine whether any of the captain's feet or arms are accessible for licking, nuzzling, or pawing. If no limbs are found, each will assume his favored position near the head of the captain; the male sitting on the captain's chest, near his face, watching for an opening to nip an exposed nose or ear, while the female assumes a full-stretch layout across the captain's face designed to stop his breathing and awaken him with a start.

If the captain tries to fake sleep and cover his head at this point, their last maneuver is the cruelest. While the female continues her attempts at suffocation, the male will circle around to where he perceives the captain's head to be buried and nuzzle under the covers for just the right tuft of the captain's hair. When a satisfactory lock is found, he will clench it tightly in his teeth and, with feet braced for the effort, pull it with maximum effort.

Your dockhands will want to take precautions if they search for them during morning hours.

After 4 p.m. and into the night, these deserters will be difficult to see or catch. Hiding and pouncing on one another occupies most of their time. However, if they are on the move, they may be tracked successfully by watching for a trail of shredded toilet paper, newspaper, or tiny bits of assorted trash. Maximum caution should be taken during these hours since a sailor's instinct for a good bar fight will overtake their inhibitions. When aware that they are being tailed, they will take cover, crouch, and bushwhack their pursuer without warning, landing a sucker's punch to the leg and bolting for a new hiding position for renewed assaults. They generally exhaust themselves with their evening grab-ass games by midnight, but often have to be kicked out of their favorite haunts and sent back to their bunks with warnings.

If you are unable to find them, just let me know and I'll continue my run south to Key West single-handed. Along the way, I may shanghai a couple of substitute crew from some dock in Virginia or North Carolina. If you do find them, please describe their condition and attitude, and I will decide whether or not to return to pick them up.

From: Dock Master, Atlantic City Marina
To: Captain, Motor Vessel *Ka Ching*
Subject: AWOL crew

Does one have a blue collar and the other a pink collar?

From: Captain, Motor Vessel *Ka Ching*
To: Dock Master, Atlantic City Marina
Subject: AWOL crew

Yes! Yes! Yes! Thank God! Please feed and comfort the little guys. They love to be held and petted. I will tie up at the next marina, rent a car, and be up there within four hours.

Thank you, thank you!

Gib arrived at Kammerman's Marina to find a pair of scared-stiff kittens that were only too pleased to leap into the rental car with Gib. When they reached *Ka Ching*, they immediately jumped back on board, made a beeline for the cat flap into the sleeping cabin, and hid under the vee-bunk.

Gib's friends heard nothing from him for the next week. I was not surprised at this hiatus because I knew how weak he was becoming and that he needed to save all of his energy for long days of travel followed by little sleep. By the time he next sent an e-mail to his list server, he had already piloted *Ka Ching* up Delaware Bay, through the C&D Canal, and all the way down Chesapeake Bay. The journey had not all been smooth sailing.

~~~~~

From: Gib Peters
To: All my family and friends
Subject: Problems on Chesapeake Bay

I reached the relative safety of the Intracoastal Waterway at Manasquan Inlet ten days ago. I was blessed by fine weather, and on the run down the Jersey coast in the open Atlantic Ocean all went well. In fact, I had time to run the film of my journey from Key West to New York backward through my mind's eye, retracing the early segments of what was to be my route back: an easy cruise down to Cape May, then a right turn and the run north through the open Delaware Bay to the C&D Canal. After that, my mind's-eye pictures changed to recall the beautifully jagged western coast of the Chesapeake Bay and the important decisions about how to navigate the bay, given wind direction, tidal speed, and the resulting wave patterns over the bay's length and width. Wave height, direction, and period would determine whether the trip down the coast was going to be a pleasant cruise or something else. It was something else!

The C&D Canal was an easy passage with no traffic and little wind. But a dark gray overcast from horizon to horizon foretold of things to come. The weather guessers reported that another cold front would roll over the area soon, led by a twenty-five-knot wind out of the west, gusts to forty, hard rain, and a low of forty-eight degrees. If I was to reach Norfolk, two hundred miles to the south, in time to make a flight to Miami to see Dr. Bradley, I'd have to push on down the Chesapeake through the rough weather.

The transit up the Chesapeake west coast, when I was on the outbound leg to New York, taught me something about the limits of my own and my vessel's ability to handle the notorious bay. I decided that the forecast didn't offer conditions that were totally impossible for us to manage, so I planned a route that would keep me hugging the windward coast where waves would be relatively easy to handle.

As the afternoon wore on and the C&D Canal faded five miles behind me, I began looking for a hurricane hole for the night on the western shore of the Chesapeake Bay. The chart showed an ideal cul-de-sac two miles south, with eight feet of depth for five hundred horizontal feet before shallowing to the beach fifty feet away in three directions. That would do nicely. I eased into the charted spot as the sun was dipping below the tree line.

Ka Ching positioned herself over a thirty-by-thirty-foot target square, and I turned the switch to release the hook. A few seconds in reverse brought the eighty feet of anchor rode snugly on a 10:1 scope, but I noticed that the anchor didn't take a bite into the bottom immediately. I had to drag it around for a few minutes in a two-hundred-foot circle before it grabbed something and finally held.

Tired, I shut down the engines, set the anchor drag alarm, fed the terrorists and myself, and crashed into bed.

The wind did indeed pick up around midnight with strong prestorm gusts. *Ka Ching* turned her nose into the wind, tugged and bobbed at her tether, but behaved well. The wind brought with it a hard-driven, noisy rain that lasted until sometime in the early morning hours. I don't understand the psychology of it, but the more turbulent it is outside, the happier I am in my warm and cozy cocoon inside. I smiled contentedly in the direction of a ball of fur wedged against my knee and went back to sleep.

My first clue that something was amiss was a morning glance out the window to see that the beach had moved a quarter of a mile further away from me than where I had left it the night before. A quick trip to the bridge in my skivvies and a check on the Garmin map verified that *Ka Ching* had dragged her anchor over what must have been a flat stone bottom for a distance of almost five hundred yards into deep water. The alarm hadn't gone off, and my confidence in the drag alarm that I had set for two hundred feet plummeted.

The GPS track showed that *Ka Ching* had dragged her hook neatly down the center of the only path possible without grounding. Was that just dumb luck or were all those prayers offered by my friends working? Whichever it was, the morning's excitement was just a harbinger of things yet to come. The overcast sky looked a bit angrier than it had the afternoon before. I turned up the thermostat a notch for a comfortable but bouncy breakfast in the cabin and turned to channel 3 for the local marine weather forecast.

"West winds at twenty-five knots with gusts to forty into the afternoon, changing to north at twenty and gusts to thirty around midnight."

That meant that the low-pressure cell that was moving from west to east would be passing me to the south, and the pressure would rise tomorrow. Better weather ahead; all I had to do today was hug the western shore as I had planned the afternoon before.

"Let's get under way, guys. Take your El Gato Siesta position in your bunks and come up to see me when your furry butts need a stretch."

The first ten miles over the next hour were uneventful, except for the occasional rain shower. The second hour had the wind begin shifting to the south and the waves picking up in a new, bow-on direction. As long as the wind held to that direction, the waves, now two to three feet, weren't all that bothersome. The head-on encounters resulted in a tolerable fore-and-aft pitch but not the head-whipping side-to-side rotation that is so uncomfortable for me on the bridge of *Ka Ching*.

But by noon, the weather guessers came under suspicion when the wind completely reversed direction from the west to east. It now had the full width of the Chesapeake Bay to build up three- to four-foot waves before they found me dodging down the western coast.

As luck would have it, there were no obvious hidey-holes on the western shore into which I could quickly dodge. I was committed to suffering the four-foot broadsides every three seconds and the resulting heavy rolling motion of my vessel for another twenty miles before I would reach the nearest safe harbor. As the side-to-side rotation increased, I began to hear the thudding and crashing of "stuff" below in the cabin that was left adrift or poorly secured. I worried about Faith and Hope being in the line of fire of heavy books in the vee-bunks, but they would have to figure out by themselves where to wedge their furry butts for the duration, out of the line of fire.

Ka Ching's center of gravity is somewhere near the water line amidships. That's safe enough, unless she pitched up to a ridiculous eighty or ninety degrees. We were topping now at around thirty-five degrees of rotation, although when the gusts were synched with a broadside, she would take a forty-degree roll that had the capacity to cause my cheeks to squeeze together around the seat cushion in a self-preserving grip.

I changed to a course that would keep the waves at a forty-five-degree angle off my port bow to minimize pitching, rolling, and yawing—a course that was taking me away from safe harbor, now fifteen miles off my starboard beam. I braced my feet against the helm, reached back for a tight grip on the stainless bar that runs behind my chair, and locked my elbows straight to stay in the chair. This prevented my body from slopping out of the chair like a wet noodle.

Under other circumstances, I would have been frightened. Instead, the emotion I felt was "wonder." Wonder at how the weather had changed so quickly, wonder at how *Ka Ching* was behaving and what her real limits were, wonder about whether my strategy for navigating the onslaught was sound, and finally wonder about how long my arm strength would last to keep me in my chair and *Ka Ching* under control. Wonder and exhilaration, but no fear.

Two hours later, the wind abated gradually, the waves lost their white tops, and *Ka Ching* behaved acceptably under the new heading to safe harbor. The hook was firmly in good holding ground, the cabin resembled a tornado track, and Hope and

Faith risked a peek from under my vee-bunk comforter. Was it luck again this time? I don't think so. Someone else is clearly aboard *Ka Ching* with us. And he had a final test in mind before I escaped the Chesapeake Bay Challenge.

Gib

~~~~~

That night, Gib slept like a baby, exhausted but proud that he had weathered the storm. However, when he woke the next morning, the weather continued to be bad—windy with high waves. His battle with the bay was far from over.

From: Gib Peters
To: All my family and friends
Subject: Near-disaster on Chesapeake Bay—the hazards of the sea

This morning, the wind was out of the west, leaving the west shoreline free of heavy seas that must be pounding the east shore by now. After listening to the weather guessers about what the day was likely to bring, I determined that the west shore down to the Potomac River would allow me to trace a route to a new anchorage fifty miles south in easy seas. It wasn't long into the run that the weather guessers changed their minds and warned that a wind shift could be expected later in the afternoon.

They were wrong again. It had already changed before I heard their report. With the wind out of the east, the west shore was kicking up quickly as the growing waves found the shallows over which I was running. I checked for a heading to my hurricane hole, now some twenty-five miles off my starboard bow, and eased the helm to the right. *Ka Ching* turned obediently to her new heading and seemed as eager as I to find an easy anchorage. But she wasn't happy. My new course put the seas on my port quarter, which resulted in a different kind of strain on *Ka Ching*. As a three- or four-foot wave washes under and lifts her stern, the stern wants to slide off the leading edge of the wave and catch up with the bow, yawing her badly to one side or the other. It takes an immediate and full helm correction to limit the yaw and hopefully keep the bow somewhere downwind and "ahead" of the stern.

So, as strong legs and feet were doing their dance over the helm, when I was about five miles into the twenty-mile journey to my sanctuary, the starboard engine suddenly faded a trifle, but then came back to life and continued to purr along. It's an unsettling moment when an engine stutters that's well known to pilots flying over water in an airplane with wheels; it's called "automatic rough." But this time I was sure it wasn't my imagination. A moment later and fully galvanized by the power fade, I watched the starboard engine's rpm drop slowly toward idle and then slump to a dead stop. The port engine continued to purr, but I was now fully alarmed. Several attempts to restart the starboard engine proved futile.

Resigned to relying now on a single engine, I turned the dead engine ignition to off, shifted the transmission to neutral, and began running down a mental checklist of possibilities for the unexpected shutdown. The port engine continued to run smoothly. Having watched the gradual, anemic failure of the starboard engine, my best guess was that the cause was fuel starvation rather than ignition or mechanical failure.

Each engine is fed by its own one-hundred-gallon tank under the afterdeck, but the fuel level for the starboard tank indicated around half of a tank remaining. That very gauge had been acting up lately, "snapping" from empty to some other level as if there were a shorted electrical connection to the fuel-level sensor. That pointed to an empty tank and a false reading. I wasn't entirely satisfied with that explanation because, after some 2,500 miles of filling and burning, I had developed a pretty good feel for how much fuel I should have in the tank by miles traveled.

Then the port engine quit! Not suddenly, but preceded by weak little coughs, just like the starboard engine twenty minutes before. The silence was shocking. My brain just didn't want to acknowledge that it could happen, but eventually it had to. And I needed to get at least one engine running before I drifted into shoaling water downwind.

I turned the second ignition to off and with great anxiety watched the sea and wind to see how *Ka Ching* would behave without power and adrift. In a minute or two she made it clear how! She would take the sea and wind that were still coming from the east . . . broadside! She rose and fell over each three-foot wave that passed beneath her, forcing her ten-foot beam into a sloppy and sickening roll. The GPS reported that we were moving about three knots over the ground, pushed by both wind and tide in the general direction of our previous heading, but toward a shoaling bar about four miles distant to the right. I had a little over an hour before trouble really began knocking on the hull.

Having put fuel starvation at the top of the list of possible ailments for the starboard engine, I had to conclude that the same problem ailed the port engine. "Impossible," I thought. But how could that be if both fuel gauges reported half tanks remaining? Bad fuel? Contamination? Water in the fuel? Water in the fuel, yes! Let's move that one to the top of the list and figure out how to safely remove the hatch covers and get to the water-fuel separators.

I swung the captain's chair to the left and felt a sharp pain through my shoulders and back. I had been gripping the stainless-steel rail along the back of the chair to hold myself in the chair with such intensity that my body ached from the effort. I hadn't been aware of the strain until I tried to work my way out of the chair and down the bridge ladder. This was not going to be fun. When I am at quiet anchor and busy in the cabin on some project or other, my diminishing physical strength often leads to an experiment of some kind to find a "work-around" solution for the new limitation. The work-around to get my tired body into position to check for water in the fuel under these conditions, and within an hour, was going to have to pop out of a lamp, cross its arms, and say: "You have three wishes, Master."

My task now was to move the three heavy hatch covers to the engines while Ka Ching rolled broadside over four-foot waves. I had to plan the move of each hatch cover carefully to drag it off its gutters and onto temporary bedding. There were three of them; each around sixty pounds. I cleared the afterdeck of the cat-litter box, rocking chair, fenders, and odds and ends, which left what appeared to be enough space for the covers when removed. I then braced myself carefully and timed the next move for a moment when the deck was level, and dragged the first hatch back into the space I had made for it. It seemed to remain in place through the rolls, so I went back for number two. Decent timing and careful sliding had both numbers two and three in a pile, leaving the engine compartment open for the next step.

I let myself down gingerly into the bilge and reached for the first filter. While I could get my hands around it, I wasn't able to turn it off. Three months ago it would have spun off with a strong one-handed grip. Not now! A bit frustrated, I turned to the second filter and gave it my soft-handed twist. It moved, and I was able to drop it off its mount. But setting it on the pitching deck while I hoisted myself out of the bilge was out of the question. I'd have to figure out how to twist my legs and body up and out, while somehow keeping a weak grip on the open filter. I had to get to a place near the side where I could safely pour the contents out into a plastic cup. In that way I could tell if there was water in the fuel. But as I struggled to roll my body out of the bilge, the filter slipped my grip and fell into the bilge, spilling the contents. Water or gas? There was now no way to find out. If I had just spilled gas in the bilge, my problems were now compounded. If water, my problems were nearly resolved.

It took five minutes to get into the cabin, get the bottle of liquid detergent, and pour it into the bilge over the muck sloshing about under the engines. That done, I crawled into a new hole to get to a seawater cock and flood the bilge, fore and aft. Twenty minutes later the bilge pumps had drained the sloshing mixture into the sea along with a cup of foaming biodegradable detergent.

A full half hour had passed, and I was becoming increasingly concerned about shoaling water downwind. And I was no further ahead to getting the engine restarted than I was when I turned off the second ignition. I spun the now-empty water separation filter back onto its mount and began a hunt for the filter wrench that I "knew" I stowed aboard *Ka Ching* in Key West before I left.

Ten minutes later I spied it under the starboard gas tank, just out of reach! In exasperation I lay as flat I could make myself in the slippery bilge, and by great good luck a sudden roll moved the wrench into my reach. Another prayer answered. I grabbed it and dragged my body as quickly as I could over the rolling deck to the engine compartment. I had very little time to get the starboard filter off and determine what it held. It turned off easily with the help of the wrench.

I placed it carefully into a nest made from a towel bunched up on the deck and hoisted myself out. The first pour of liquid into the transparent cup showed no layers, but the liquid I saw was very dirty. I was halfway convinced now that I was looking at water because gas doesn't hold dirt in suspension that way. The second and last pour into the transparent cup showed a layer: an eighth of an inch of amber gas on top, and three inches of dirty water beneath it.

That was it, then! Fuel starvation due to water contamination.

I spun on the second filter and scrambled to get the port hatch back on and replaced the ladder to the bridge. I reached my captain's chair and turned briefly to the GPS map to see how far I had drifted over the past hour. I was alarmed to find that I was already over a four-foot shoal with just two feet of clearance between the bottom and the propellers. I quickly pumped the starboard throttle and cranked the starter. The engine wouldn't catch, and the depth went to three feet with one foot under the propellers.

After fifteen seconds of cranking, when enough new gas filled the filter and found its way to the carburetor, the starboard engine coughed and caught. I didn't bother trying to restart the port engine; I didn't have time. I carefully put the transmission into reverse and turned the helm left while bringing the rpm up to 1,200.

Slowly the stern overcame the push of the waves and began to creep away from the shallow water. Three feet, four feet, six feet—I was home free. A fifteen-second crank of the port engine was similarly rewarded with a cough and a rumble. Both engines now rumbled contentedly and showed no more signs of sucking down anything but pure gas.

Three hours later, safely tucked away in my hurricane hole, I puzzled about the problem. Water it was. But where did it come from? Almost always, water builds up in gas tanks as a result of condensation caused by the periodic heating and cooling of the air around and in the tank.

But condensation was unlikely, because I had added an emulsifier only a week before to get rid of any pooling water at the bottom of the tanks. After I turned down the lights and climbed into bed, it came to me. Aside from condensation there were only two points of ingress for water: the filler tube and the vent tube. The filler is sealed with a cap. But each tank is fitted with an air vent at the top terminating on the side of the hull about four inches from the gunnels. I pulled myself out of my bunk, turned on the lights on the afterdeck, and leaned over the side. That was it. Each vent had a small "clamshell" deflector mounted on the hull, turned downward, which must have cupped and captured a sip of sea water from every wave on every roll throughout the day, delivering it directly into the gas tank.

The Duct Tape Consumers Council would have been proud of me. Five minutes later I had fashioned an ugly "shield and drain" for each vent to deflect and drain the seas away from the vulnerable opening.

Another victory! Through the aches and pains, sleep last night came quickly and was sweet indeed.

And to all my loved ones, sleep well.

Gib

It was hard for an amateur sailor like me to conceive how Gib, so weakened by his ALS, could steer a twenty-nine-foot motor cruiser through gales and pounding waves on Chesapeake Bay, managing both the wheel and engine controls with his legs and feet. His head rocked painfully around with each pitch and roll of the boat. And he had to feed himself by pouring four cans of liquid food into his PEG tube three times a day—if the storms gave him time to "eat." Though Iron Mike was useful for cruising in fine weather, it was useless in a storm.

From: Walter Bradley
To: Gib Peters
Subject: Near-disaster on Chesapeake Bay—the hazards of the sea

Dear Gib,

I swear that you do these things just to get us all in a panic! Your writing skills do not diminish. You clearly have the talent to make a career as a thriller writer. I am glad you survived! We all pray for fair weather and fine sailing in the coming weeks as you wend your weary way back to the home of all that is good in politics—Florida!!

Walter

While Gib was battling the seas, the country was engaged in another battle. The U.S. presidential election was being contested in Florida, "Home of the Hanging Chad."

From: Gib Peters
To: Dr. Walter Bradley
Subject: Near-disaster on Chesapeake Bay—the hazards of the sea

I stay up most of the night making lists, prioritizing them, and then selecting the adventure that will stress you guys the most. Did it work?

Gib

Amazingly, Gib and *Ka Ching* survived the pounding on Chesapeake Bay. Gib steered *Ka Ching* southward through the Great Dismal Swamp Canal into the open waters of Albemarle Sound in North Carolina. He reached the broad Pamlico River and there experienced the bloodiest part of his odyssey.

~~~~~

From: Gib Peters
To: All my family and friends
Subject: No Good Deed Goes Unpunished

The Pamlico River is a broad, slow-moving body of water, more like a miniature Chesapeake Bay at a mere five miles across. But like most broad rivers and sounds flowing into the Atlantic along the Eastern Seaboard, the Pamlico is dredged in its shallowest points for the Intracoastal Waterway, running perpendicular through it from north to south. The average depth of the ICW along the North Carolina coastline is about six feet—enough water to accommodate small private motor yachts up to fifty feet in length, tugs and barges, and most long-legged sailboats. Outside the channel, water depths are surprisingly shallow, in the range of one to four feet over vast stretches of the river.

I had just finished the southbound transit across the Pamlico River and was turning into the Goose River at green marker 6. About a hundred yards ahead and to the left of the channel, I saw two forty-foot sailboats with no sails aloft, dead in the water and obviously aground. I slowed my speed to idle as I passed, not wanting to make life even more difficult for these guys, but to my surprise the captains of both vessels were hailing me to increase my speed.

I was confused about the request, but as I passed the second boat I caught on to their hope that some heavy wakes rocking their keels might allow them to motor free of the mud and back into the channel. I waved acknowledgement and made a 180-degree turn to set up for a high-speed pass. I idled up to marker 6, turned south again, and lined up to pass within fifteen feet of their starboard beams. I added enough throttle to keep *Ka Ching* off a plane and producing the biggest wake I could manage. As I did so, the captains advanced their own engine throttles to maximum as their vessels rocked in the wake. I looked back to see how they reacted, and they signaled for another pass. Another 180 and another big-wake pass, and the second boat struggled free and moved into the channel. Encouraged, I then passed the first boat another three times with no result. The boat hadn't even rolled in the wake. It was hard aground. "Well, here's a sailor in a jam. Now what do I do?"

I pulled up close to the remaining boat and pantomimed to the captain, asking if he would like to attempt a tow. He said that he would, and I signaled him to board my boat and tend the tow line on the afterdeck, since I was single-handed. As I maneuvered my stern to his bow, he jumped aboard and one of his remaining crew tossed him a one-inch hawser. He pulled it all aboard and looked around for a cleat. Although the wind was light, the current in the river was enough to keep me busy at the controls to prevent either collision with the sailboat or grounding myself, so I didn't supervise his preparations. After all, I thought, he's the captain of his vessel, not a crew member; he should have the skills needed for a simple tow.

He made the tow line fast to one of the cleats on the starboard side of my transom and then shouted for me to "give it gas." I waved acknowledgment over my shoulder, taking his instruction to mean that we had taken a strain on the tow line and that power was now needed to move the sailboat. I added power, and *Ka Ching* leaped ahead a few feet. The line parted with a jerk and a snap. I knew right away that the line had not been straining but instead had been lying on the deck when he signaled me to "give it gas."

A bit surprised with how this captain had managed the tow line, I moved upwind, put *Ka Ching* into neutral, and went down to the deck to explain on my clipboard to him that I wanted a strain on the line before he gave me a signal to add power. He nodded that he understood, and I regained my seat on the bridge. This time I was resolved to wait until I felt the tug of the straining tow line before I added power.

I backed carefully to near the bow of the sailboat, and after three attempts the line was again caught by the captain on my afterdeck. This time I was drifting toward the same shallow water the sailboat had encountered, and I was maneuvering to avoid both his bow and the shallow water when I felt a thump and rumble from below.

The first thing I suspected was that my propellers had dug into the mud. But then I heard the captain on the afterdeck yell to me that he was unable to get the tow line free. That was when I realized that the tow line had rolled up on my propellers. I shifted to neutral and dropped down to the deck with the faint hope that I was wrong.

But what I saw confirmed the worst. The tow line was indeed straining, but on a straight line from the sailboat bow to a point under my transom. It was apparent that our good captain had made the line fast to the cleat on the stern and then dumped the entire length of the tow line over the side into the water, instead of paying it out from the deck. *Ka Ching* now trailed downstream from the sailboat. The two of us were now helpless and powerless.

And the sun was sinking quickly to the horizon.

To his credit, the captain asked if he should go over the side and cut it loose. I motioned to him to wait, that I had another idea first. Exasperated, I returned to the bridge and attempted to reverse the propellers at idle speed in hopes that the line might fall free. That was too much to expect, and the line became entangled ever more tightly in the blades as a result. Each of my shafts has a set of cutting spurs mounted just ahead of the propeller and designed to cut any lines picked up while the shafts turned. While they are quite effective for quarter- or even half-inch line, they are no match for the heavy one-inch hawser we were using for a tow line. I tried the starboard side once more and was rewarded with a "kerchunk" and a freely running starboard propeller. But the port shaft remained tight and dragged the engine to a stop when it was shifted to either forward or reverse.

I was in a pickle. I signaled to the crew of the sailboat to haul us alongside and raft us up. The captain of the grounded sailboat, realizing his error in handling the line, volunteered again to dive down to the propellers with a knife and cut the entangled line. I agreed and he stripped down.

"How cold is the water?" he asked. I checked the water temperature and scribbled "58" on my clipboard. "Geez," was all he said as he pulled on his flippers and mask. I was not confident in his judgment as a sailor, but I had to admit he had guts as a diver.

"When I get into the water, hand me a knife," he said. I went into the cabin and picked out the sharpest eight-inch cutter and took it out to where he was waiting. He nodded and I watched him step over the side and into the chilly water. The splash was immediately followed by his body erupting from the plume.

"Whaaa hooo!!" he shouted. "That's cold!"

Already stressed by the cold and shuddering uncontrollably, he reached up to me. "Gimme the knife," he sputtered. I handed it down to him handle first, and he wrenched it from my hand, nearly turning the blade into my palm as he submerged. I was a bit miffed that he wasn't a bit more careful, but understood the difficult conditions under which he was working. After only about five seconds, he emerged sputtering again, reporting that he dropped the knife and needed another. I ran into the cabin, got my next best cutter, came back to the ladder, and handed the knife down to him. He tried to raise his arm but couldn't get his elbow out of the water.

It was then that I saw a stream of blood spurting from his outreached arm. "Oh no, I'm cut, I'm cut. I can't feel my hand. My arm is numb," he screamed. I motioned for him to pull himself up the ladder, but he just screamed and watched the blood pour from a hole in his arm. He then grappled with the ladder with his right arm, but his left remained immobile and unused. On the second step up the ladder, he faltered, and I got my left fist full of T-shirt and did my best to pull him into the boat.

Blood covered both of us and most of the deck where I stood. My mind went immediately to the distress call I had heard on channel 16 about a fisherman whose arm was slashed by a barracuda. The bleeding couldn't be stopped, and the Coast Guard picked him up and moved him to a hospital just in time to save his life.

While the captain stood on the deck bleeding, I went down to the cabin and looked in the medicine cabinet for something to press against the wound. I had put in a supply of sanitary napkins for just such an emergency; I tore one open. I found him leaning on the side, shuddering uncontrollably, babbling about needing an aspirin and that he couldn't feel his fingers. I pressed the napkin hard against the wound and got his other hand to hold it while I did my best "spit-yell" for his crew on the sailboat. Getting him to keep the compress on the wound wasn't as easy as described, because the poor guy was beside himself with fear for all the blood on the deck and the loss of sensation.

Finally his crew came aboard and spotted the spray of blood over the afterdeck. One guy immediately threw up, turned around, and made his way unsteadily back to the sailboat. The other fellow was made of sterner stuff, caught on quickly, and helped get the captain into my cabin and onto a chair. I turned up the heat, pulled a blanket from the bunk, and helped his first mate throw it over his captain.

Controlling the bleeding was priority number one. He continued to say that he thought he should have aspirin, but I shook my head. The guy wasn't having a heart attack, and aspirin would only exacerbate the bleeding. He was difficult to settle down long enough to determine what kind of bleeding we were dealing with: arterial or venous.

He finally began to show signs of understanding that he needed to remain quiet and let me look at the wound. I cleaned the arm and sneaked a peek under the pads for a closer look at the wound. Surprisingly, I found the wound to be a mere one inch across and no longer bleeding! The arm however was beginning to swell badly.

He needed some good news, so I scribbled a note saying "numbness temporary, bleeding under control . . . no immediate danger." I knew I had the bleeding part right, but I didn't have a clue about the numbness. It appeared that he had cut some finger nerves, but I didn't feel that I should share that guess. He asked me if I was a doctor. I shook my head and remembered something from a captain's first aid course years before. Tell the patient that you are "medically trained and able to help." My instructor said it would calm the patient and make first aid easier to administer. I scribbled a note to this effect, and he relaxed!

My hands by now were weak and not strong enough to roll sterile gauze around the wound. The first mate took over the manual tasks, and I wrote notes. While the wound was small, it was quite deep. It appeared that the point of the knife had entered the forearm with a stabbing movement and nearly exited on the other side. His uncontrolled cold-induced spasms in the water probably had the knife slashing wildly about under the boat. It was only sheer luck that he hadn't stuck the knife into his body or cut an artery in his neck.

He continued to settle down; his color returned, the trembling stopped, and he shed the blanket. It was pushing eighty-five degrees in the cabin, and it appeared that the bleeding would not restart as long the gauze wrapping remained in place. If I could have talked, I would have called the Coast Guard at that point to ask for assistance. I suggested by a note that he or his first mate give them a call, but the captain declined, saying he felt better and that he would see how he felt in a half hour or so. In the meantime we decided to put a call in to Tow Boat U.S., something we should have done before I offered to tow them free.

After a few minutes, towing assistance from Belhaven, fifteen miles north, was under way to our position. I suggested that he should be airlifted to a hospital, but he again declined, now saying that he didn't want to leave his boat with an inexperienced crew at night and that he thought he should anchor nearby and wait for morning. I tried one more time, writing a note saying that he should see a doctor tonight and get a tetanus shot. But he declined again.

Two hours later, the twenty-five-foot all-red Tow Boat U.S. showed up, the guy having located us with a powerful spotlight. We told him that I needed a tow to a repair facility and the sailboat needed a tow off the mud. He told the sailboat crew to cut me loose and let me drift downstream. After pulling the sailboat free he would pick me up and take me under tow. I didn't like the idea of drifting uncontrolled, so I started the starboard engine that had the usable propeller and pushed off.

It was pitch-black now, so I picked out a five-hundred-foot-diameter circle upwind of the two other boats and began making idle-speed circles in deep water on my GPS map. Before long I saw the sailboat move to an anchorage a half mile away, but I couldn't see the tow boat or its lights.

I soon found it.

He had moved directly ahead of my vessel without lights, without radio coordination or other warning, and had squatted directly in my path, quite invisible. WHAMM! My bow ran up and nearly through his forward railing, putting a nice series of deep gouges on *Ka Ching*'s painted gel coat on the starboard bow.

"Sorry, Captain, I didn't know you were under power," came a voice out of the dark.

"Yeah sure, Captain, I'm upwind, up current, and I've been circling with every light burning for the last twenty minutes . . . tell me about it," I thought.

He finally got the bridle on, took the strain, and moved his speed up to seven knots for the two-hour tow back to Belhaven.

The next morning I put a call into my insurance company to send an appraiser. As I write today, I am thirteen days behind schedule and the insurance company is down $7,000 in shaft and strut repairs. I don't have a clue where the sailboats are and how the captain is doing, but I'm wondering about the truth of the old axiom "No good deed goes unpunished." I'm tempted to subscribe to it after my Pamlico River experience, but instead I've printed out a new one and pasted it to my galley fridge: "No offer of a tow will go unpunished."

Gib

I was very worried when I read this e-mail, not just for Gib in his ever-more disabled state but also for the sailboat captain with the stab wound in his arm. The rapid swelling meant that the bleeding was arterial and that blood was beginning to accumulate in the tissues of the arm. The captain had cut an artery in his arm and probably some nerves as well. The bleeding shut down because the artery went into spasm with the cold, but his refusal to go to the nearest hospital was foolhardy. I later contacted the sailboat captain and learned that he did eventually go to a hospital; he was lucky enough to have survived without major consequences.

Tow Boat U.S. took *Ka Ching* back to Belhaven, a small town of less than two thousand souls with a snug harbor, relying on tourism, fishing, boating, and wildlife. Once more *Ka Ching* was in dry dock, this time to repair the port-side propeller and prop shaft. Gib was back in North Carolina, where he was without cell phone coverage. Since he clearly was not going anywhere soon, he typed up and faxed a letter to Marcia giving her the short version of the tale of the two grounded sailboats. He told her that he was safe in the boatyard and asked her to let everyone know that he would not be able to contact them till he had cell phone coverage again.

In his fax to Marcia, Gib admitted for the first time that his condition was beginning to cause even him concern: "My hands and arms are getting weaker, as expected. If the repairs are done quickly, I think I will be able to get home without a problem." The unspoken message was that he was starting to think that he might not make it back to Key West.

Nearly 1,100 nautical miles still stretched between Gib and Key West. Repairs to the damaged struts, propeller, and prop shaft required that *Ka Ching* be hoisted out of the water and put up on blocks once more. Getting the parts and completing the repairs took over two weeks.

While *Ka Ching* was still in the yard in Belhaven, Gib flew down to Miami for his research trial appointment with me. It was clear that his ALS was progressing rapidly. He had lost another ten pounds in the last two months and was having difficulty turning over in bed and dressing. His legs were beginning to show some signs of weakness, making him increasingly at risk of falling and slowing his movements around the boat. Because his right hand was continuing to weaken, his writing on the clipboard was now illegible. However, he could still type on the computer with his left index finger. It was fortunate that he never lost that ability!

On November 12, with a repaired boat and renewed determination, Gib left Belhaven on the Intracoastal Waterway. He kept his speed between eight and ten knots and traveled long hours, relying more and more on Iron Mike to steer *Ka Ching*. All he wanted was to get the trip over as rapidly as possible. The last phase of his odyssey was taking on an atmosphere of desperation.

More than two hundred bridges cross the Atlantic Intracoastal Waterway (ICW) between the Manasquan Inlet in New Jersey and Key West at the southern tip of Florida. Many have such low clearance that boats cannot pass without the bridge being opened. In the stretch from Portsmouth, Virginia, to Miami, there are over seventy such low-clearance bridges. Gib managed to navigate through all these using one of several strategies. From the charts and tables he could find the scheduled times when the bridge opened; he could act out a vigorous pantomime of his needs when he came into sight of the bridge master; or he could use his computer voice simulator to call over the radio.

Other bridges on the ICW have a clearance of more than fifty feet, and *Ka Ching* easily navigated under them. Gib and his able-bodied feline crew had been under every one of these high bridges going both north- and southbound without a problem—until they came to the Atlantic Beach Bridge in North Carolina on November 13. The following e-mail, published in two parts in the Sunday *Key West Citizen* on December 19 and December 26, 2004, were the final installments in the series about Gib's odyssey.

From: Gib Peters
To: All my family and friends
Subject: Grief and a Bridge in North Carolina

I struggled through an emotionally wrenching day yesterday. I lost Faith, one of my stalwart feline crew. The morning started as one of the nicest of the trip: a bright blue sky from horizon to horizon, calm winds, and mirrored serpentine rivers winding their way through flat South Carolina coastal marshes. It's surreal to see a large, fully rigged sailboat a half mile away moving silently over table-flat fields of grass. Life was good.

A high, graceful concrete bridge was looming ahead with tiny cars hurrying about their business in both directions. Hope and Faith hate bridges of any description because of their threatening shadows and the roaring echo of *Ka Ching*'s engines off the bridge fenders as we pass beneath. A couple of hundred feet from a bridge, they suddenly awaken to the threat and launch themselves to a place of cover under the helm or in the cabin.

As we approached this particular monster, Hope bolted off my lap and scurried to his "special safe place" under the helm. Faith, who prefers to find a lookout position somewhere around the lower decks, apparently saw the bridge coming from her chosen spot on the starboard side just below the bridge. I couldn't see her, but I guessed where she was from the sudden, desperate scratching of small claws trying to get a grip on the slippery gel coat sides of the boat.

I've often imagined and feared that sound as the signal of a cat overboard, but never heard it until now. A small but distinctive splash followed. I immediately jumped out of my chair and leaned over the starboard side for a fast scan of the water for a cat bobbing in the wake.

Nothing.

I slapped the engine throttles down to idle and again intently studied the water immediately behind and to the sides of *Ka Ching* for a distance of thirty yards or so.

No cat. Just boiling, brown river water from angrily turning blades beneath my vessel. With the engine transmissions moved to neutral and with *Ka Ching* drifting in a narrow channel under the bridge, I climbed down to the afterdeck and focused every sense at my command over the sides and directly aft for a tiny head.

Still nothing.

But farther back, from around a bend a quarter mile back, I caught sight of the heavily laden barge and tug that I had passed

just minutes before. The barge was plowing the water into a sloping bulge from its blunt bow and moving with heavy purpose
toward me. Any more time spent drifting in the narrow channel
under the bridge was a recipe for a yet bigger disaster. I reluctantly remounted my chair and pulled ahead and to the right of
the channel to a place where I wouldn't risk a collision. *Ka Ching*
settled to a stop in ten feet of water, allowing me a few minutes to
rethink the problem. Maybe Faith made it to the cabin after all!

I dropped down to the cabin and went to the vee-bunk first.
I tore the unkempt comforter off, reached into the back of the
bookcases, into the drawers, and in every other hidey-hole where
she's been found before. My fear heightened as I moved to the
galley, the head, the counters, drawers, cabinets, deck holes, and
other special cat nooks. Still no sign of Faith. On the afterdeck,
a look around the dock boxes, rocking chair, and trashcan produced nothing.

She did go over the side.

By this time *Ka Ching* was drifting slowly into shallow water,
having been nudged by the pressure of the barge that had just
passed. But the river northward was now clear for a careful
search. I climbed the bridge ladder with newfound strength and
with urgent purpose.

As I turned *Ka Ching* back under the bridge, I remembered the
two-knot current that was running north and the possibility that
it had swept her upstream further than I initially estimated. With
renewed hope and a growing fervent wish to see her small head
bobbing in the channel, I headed north at five knots with a steady
visual sweep of the water ahead. Apart from an upturned brown
beer bottle and a piece of knobby driftwood, I saw nothing that
could have been a struggling cat.

Cats can swim, by the way. They dislike water and only reluctantly get near it. But once in the water they can swim dog-paddle

like black Labs for hours or even days at a time. I heard about a sailboat in the Florida Gulf Stream that recovered a swimming cat far from land and with no other boat in sight. This continued to feed my withering hope for her recovery, though it was tempered by recalling that the Gulf Stream is seventy to eighty degrees year-round, while my keel thermometer read fifty-eight degrees. Faith's chances would grow slim as the cold water sucked the heat from her tiny body.

Time was running out.

I was growing feverish in my luckless search but tried to remain disciplined about the ever-widening search pattern. I thought, "Maybe I somehow missed her in my initial search of the boat. That has to be it. I've covered almost a full mile of water in two sweeps. If she was on the surface, I would have seen her." Having talked myself into the possibility, I found another deep water pocket off the channel and left *Ka Ching* to drift while I did a more thorough search of the entire vessel. This time I started on the bridge, checking every nook and cranny with a flashlight and with blind grabs into awkward holes.

Down on the lower deck, I did an inch-by-inch, overturn-everything examination of the cabin, the head, vee-bunk, rope locker, fuse compartment, drawers, cabinets, shelves, laundry bags, atop the printer, on the radio, behind escutcheons, the bilge areas, and even inside the refrigerator. Again on the afterdeck I tore apart the tool chest, dock boxes, life jacket stowage, trash can, paint locker, oil stowage, and peered under the gunnels while spit-mumbling nice "Come-here-kitty" noises all the time. Not a hair. My last desperate probe was in the engine compartment. God knows, the engine and generator spaces would be the worst place for a cat to stow away for any length of time, because of the high risk of physical injury, carbon monoxide poisoning, and heat prostration.

But even as I uncovered the spaces, exposing possible hiding spots, I knew there was little chance of her being there, dead or alive, because she had been romping around the deck after I sealed up the deck that morning. Nothing. Not a clue. Faith was gone, and the empty, gnawing feeling in my stomach was palpable.

I was crushed.

She must have succumbed immediately to the cold or the shock of being ducked under water for the first time in her life, and simply drowned. Inhaling a teacup of water when she first hit would have resulted in negative buoyancy immediately, and the turbulence would have kept her down. Then there were the barge and tug. Her chances of surviving their passage were close to zero.

I reluctantly climbed to the bridge for one last attempt to sweep the mile-long search segment, but this time with special attention to the shorelines. My eyes welled with tears as much from emotion as from the strain as I tried to imagine what a cold, wet cat on a rock would look like. What did I do wrong? What should have I done better to protect her?

Several months ago I gave up trying to keep the cats off the bow and the gunnels. They were maturing fast and becoming headstrong about their right to be cats. So I hung two "cat overboard ladders" made of plastic netting from each side of the stern platform, hoping that if they fell overboard they would have a chance to get back aboard. I fully intended to get them into the water for swimming lessons and some "cat ladder" instruction, but the water temperatures were slipping below sixty, and I didn't have the heart to put them over the side. Not that the ladders would have helped them while cruising at seven knots. They were meant for use during overnight anchorages, where they loved to romp and skylark around topside until midnight or so. For underway cat-overboard drills, I had put together a "cat retriever" by attaching a lobster net to the end of my ten-foot boat hook. I never used it, but it was snugly stowed and ready for use under the starboard gunnel.

Where did I screw up?

I had the same parental problems while raising these two young kittens in a dangerous environment as I had with my children as they pushed the limits while growing up. I tried to restrict and train them, but eventually learned to soften my limits as I saw them handle the new responsibility with caution and apparent care. Even after the AWOL incident, I found myself allowing Hope and Faith to roam around marina docks near the boat at sundown, because they unerringly returned around midnight looking for a place to curl up under my comforter. I never slept well on those nights until I heard the cat flap swing open and shut. Twice.

The shoreline search was completed, the water scans had proved unproductive, and an intensive search of my vessel had turned up nothing.

My cat and friend, Faith, was gone.

I fell into a nightmare-like, self-flagellating depression, imagining what her last moments must have been like. Unable to grip the side of the boat, plunging suddenly into a cold swirling water, and seeing the only sanctuary she had ever known move down the river with a steady, unconcerned rumble; how terrified she must have been. I could only hope that she had gone down quickly and hadn't suffered being hurt by my propellers or later by the tug and barge chewing their way down the river.

It was over, then! There was nothing to do but move on. And so I did.

As the afternoon passed I put as much distance as I could between me and that damned bridge, thinking about life and death from a different perspective. The emptiness in my gut was so real and so deep that I was startled. I tried to plumb the depths of my grief, pitting reason against emotion. "It's just a cat, Gibber; and it wasn't your fault." "Yeah, but I loved her," I answered myself. "She would push her head into my hand for a rub, she talked to me with her squeaky little voice, and she crept onto my lap and gave me a paw to hold while I was reading." The longer this one-sided conversation went on, the deeper became the despair and the more tangible the grief.

Then it struck me: The roles had suddenly reversed. It was not I who was dying and leaving others to live on. It was I who was living on after losing someone I loved. The irony only brought a new level of distress to the day's experience. Does my family feel the emptiness about my dying as I am feeling for the death of Faith? Is this the emptiness, the anguish and helplessness they are feeling this very moment? I imagined that it must be so and was numbed by my newest understanding of the effects of my disease. How much more terrible it is for them than for me. I had no idea how they must be feeling until this moment.

I've got the easy part. Facing death as a near-at-hand, slam-dunk certainty changes the zeitgeist of one's time remaining. The initial shock of it passes quickly. Then you just move the horizon closer and get all your unfinished business finished. For those who are about to be left behind, it is, I understand now, far more devastating. Marcia is so strong. But I think now she is strong for me. I had no idea just how deep the hurt must be for her, nor any appreciation for what she must be feeling.

And what about my kids? They join me in making light of my spit-mumble speech and my awkward hands, and in so doing, tell me that they're OK; that they are coping. But I think now that their awkward attempts at humor are covering for their distress. Until that North Carolina bridge, I hadn't really guessed what my family must be feeling and how well their cover is working. The emptiness I was then feeling for the loss of a cat could only be multiplied by some exponential number for the certain loss of their dad. I learned a stunning lesson today.

It was around 5 p.m., just fifteen minutes before sunset. It's later than I usually run, but I couldn't bear going below at the usual 3 p.m. and not having Faith nuzzling my hand for an early dinner. The quicker I could just wash up, drain four cans of formula into my feeding tube, and get to sleep, the better. I found a nice anchorage, listened to the clatter of the anchor chain rolling over the pulpit, and felt it grab firmly into a soft, mud bottom. The noisy anchor chain is an automatic alert for the crew to get out of their bunks and begin the afternoon watch for dolphin, fish, and birds around the anchorage and begin pestering me for a dish of meat mush. This was not going to be easy today.

I backed down the first steps of the bridge ladder and froze: Hope was at the foot of the ladder in the middle of a full-body stretch, with his rear end arched high and his front legs reaching out flat on the deck. But Hope had on a pink collar! Faith's collar! "What the—!"

I quickly looked up under the helm to see if Hope had beaten me down the ladder. He had not. I was looking straight into his huge post-siesta yawn at the top of the ladder and at his blue collar. I had two cats aboard! Two cats!! Nobody was missing, nobody died, everybody was present and accounted for and casually getting ready for evening chow. I nearly fell down the last two steps in an awkward attempt to gather up Faith for a grateful, tearful embrace.

But as she has grown heavier, my arms have grown weaker. She must have wondered why I was pulling her rear end up into the air and leaving her front paws planted on the deck. So I just lay down on the deck, collected her to me for a long embrace, and launched into a happy spit-mumble lecture about coming out of hiding when I made a certain distressed, nasal-sounding snort. I was ecstatic. The hurt and the emptiness evaporated, the depression and the grief disappeared, and in their place was the boundless happiness of being together again.

But as thrilled and grateful as I was, my thoughts kept drifting back to my family. I was seeing them for the first time through a newfound lens of understanding. I was seeing their hidden suffering, grief, and anguish for their loss to come for the first time. In a flash, I saw both sides of grief. Theirs is indescribably hard. I'll make it through just fine. It isn't I who is brave, inspirational, or remarkable in any way, cruising through rivers and bays. Those who love me are all of that and so much more. It is THEY who deserve MY attention, care, and comfort through these hard times. What I need to do now is go home and be at hand as they cope with the emptiness they must feeling.

Yes, I've got it straight now. Faith taught me that.

Gib

~~~~~

On November 15, at the end of a long day, Gib brought *Ka Ching* into Hinckley Yacht Marina, the scene of so much frustration back in July when he had tried to get Westerbeke Corporation to repair his generator. He now needed a replacement riser on one of his Chevy 350-cubic-inch V8 engines. He had already e-mailed Dustin Hartley and Nancy Veenstra to let them know that he was coming and what he wanted. He indicated that he was in a great hurry to get back to Key West. They recognized the reason as soon as they saw how much he had deteriorated since July. Hinckley's mechanics completed the repairs in record time, and *Ka Ching* cruised out of Savannah River and southward on the morning of November 18.

Now surviving on mental energy alone, with his motor neurons continuing to die and his body to weaken, Gib pushed *Ka*

Ching and himself as much as he dared. On November 20, he arrived in Jacksonville, Florida, and was at Daytona Beach marina on the afternoon of November 22. Kim brought her young children to see him one last time. She was shocked to see just how much Gib had deteriorated since their time together in New York. She cried afterward, realizing he had very little time left.

On the evening of Monday, November 22, Gib dropped anchor out of the channel, a short distance off Titusville Municipal Marina. The next day he took the dinghy into the marina to meet George and the family, who had come to take him to Key West for Thanksgiving. Mike, Lisa and her family, and Kim and her family drove Gib, plus the two cats in carriers on top of one of the cars, 375 miles to the family home in Key West. They had a wonderful Thanksgiving, and Gib rested at home for the weekend. On Monday, November 29, George drove Gib, Faith, and Hope back to *Ka Ching* in Titusville.

Gib was still thinking he could take the cross-Florida waterway to St. Petersburg and visit Wally Dutcher. However, in a flurry of e-mails, Wally and Marcia persuaded him that this was sheer foolishness.

Gib set off in his dinghy from his anchorage in Titusville on the morning of December 1. To the east, on one of the deserted islands that he named Dylan Key, after one of his grandsons, he buried "treasure" so that his "grands and great-grands" could discover it at some time in the future. The treasure consisted of things of no monetary worth in themselves, but Gib believed that they would be of immeasurable value to his descendants. He recorded the spot on the island with photographs and a map that Marcia still keeps for her children and grandchildren.

On the evening of December 2, Gib anchored in Hobe Sound, Florida, between Stuart and Jupiter, where the Intracoastal Waterway runs only four hundred yards from a beautiful beach bordering the Atlantic Ocean.

From: Gib Peters
To: All my family and friends
Subject: Report

Just a quick report to friends and family about my progress down the East Coast. I anchored last night in a little cove in Hobe Sound, about eighty miles north of Miami. And it's a glorious Florida morning. My travel goal today will be to anchor for the night in a tiny wide place in the ICW called Lettuce Lake in Pompano. It's getting tough to find any kind of isolation, deep water, and swing room off the waterway because of the heavy residential building all along the ICW in this stretch. Civilization!

I'm anxious to get home to squeeze my bride. She has been tolerant of my fantasy trip for seven months and altogether supportive of the huge gasoline bills that keep showing up in the mailbox. She's my woman; I love her for all of that and for many other reasons.

I'm anxious because I have to admit to having considerable difficulty with sharply diminished strength in the arms, neck, shoulders, and hands. Although I've been on 3,200 calories a day, I am down to 164 pounds from two hundred-plus a year ago. My muscles are wasting quickly, and the frustration with simple tasks using my arms and hands is dominating my day. It's time to go home.

Let me finally apologize for the short report; it's all one-finger typing now. For the blabbermouth writer that I am, that's the toughest part. More later.

Love to all,
Gib

I thought it unlikely that Gib would make the last 260 miles to Key West. His arms were useless, he was struggling with typing with only his left index finger, and he was only able to hold the PEG tube funnel to feed himself with extraordinary trick maneuvers. His breathing was weak. I feared that before reaching Key West he would die either of respiratory failure or of one too many falls.

Gib's son-in-law George was also fairly certain that Gib would not get to Key West. He discussed Plan B with Marcia: They would drive to wherever the crisis occurred and collect him, worrying later about getting the boat back to Key West.

Determined, Gib hung on for a last desperate effort to get to Key West before he collapsed. He pushed the throttles forward with his foot and had *Ka Ching* up to fifteen knots, disregarding the "Caution! Manatees" speed zones and the risk of getting oil in the bilge. He was going home—do or die.

On December 3 he traveled over sixty miles and anchored in Pompano, among the $5 million homes and fifty-foot luxury cruisers that cost almost as much. On December 4 he covered nearly seventy miles, motoring past Fort Lauderdale and Miami, to anchor for the night between Totten Key and Ocean Reef Club, just north of Key Largo.

The next day, he traveled another sixty miles to anchor that evening on the Florida Bay side of Duck Key. Despite his weakness and the desperate need to get home, he forced his failing body to take the dinghy over to Channel Key to bury another cache of "treasure" for his descendants.

Key West was still over sixty miles away, but Gib thought he might be able to make it there without having to stop for another night. He rose early on the morning of December 6, 2004, rushed through his early morning routine, and set off with the vision of Marcia and his home in Key West in his mind's eye.

Late that afternoon Gib turned the wheel of *Ka Ching* to port to enter Riviera Channel. He was half a mile from home. Gib was sitting back in his captain's chair, steering the boat with his feet as he had done for most of the four thousand miles that he had traveled in the last seven months. Deftly he spun the wheel and reversed the engines, turning *Ka Ching* 180 degrees to back her into the dock at his house. Marcia and their friends jumped onto the boat to secure the lines. Gib's legs were still reasonably good, and he insisted on getting off the boat under his own steam.

Whether it was because he knew that he must stink of sweat, gasoline, and seawater, or whether it was out of sheer exuberance at having completed his marathon odyssey to New York and back, we shall never know. But for whatever reason, his first action on reaching his dock was to dive into the swimming pool.

This was foolhardy, to say the least! Gib had not taken a swim during the whole of his journey and clearly didn't realize the changes that had occurred to his body during that time. He had lost his ability to use his arms to swim; he could not hold up his head to breathe; and his mouth and throat were so weak that he could not stop water from going into his lungs. He began to splutter violently and sink to the bottom of the pool. He would have drowned if several friends had not jumped in and pulled him out.

Once he was seated in his own deck chair between *Ka Ching* at the dock and the patio doors of his house, Gib burst into spluttering laughter. Soon everyone was laughing, cheering, and clapping him on the back. Champagne corks popped, and they toasted him for the successful completion of his unbelievable odyssey.

After all the exertions of the past seven months, especially the strain of the last week, Gib was completely and utterly exhausted. Marcia helped him up to bed, accompanied by his two cats, Faith and Hope. By now, Gib was unable to turn over in bed, so he slept in a fetal position with the two cats curled up around him.

When Marcia was sure he was asleep, she went downstairs to join their friends. Together with Dick Mooney, she went to look at *Ka Ching*. They were amazed at the remarkably good condition of the boat. Despite his disabilities, Gib had kept *Ka Ching* in good mechanical repair, apart from a few places that needed a lick of paint. On the other hand, with regard to tidiness and aroma, the less said the better.

From: Gib Peters
To: All my family and friends
Subject: Home at last!

Don't anybody cash in my insurance policy . . . I'm home! I spent my last evening a hundred yards from Channel Key, just north of Duck Key. It was so good to be in familiar Keys water; even *Ka Ching* behaved differently. That was Sunday night. On Monday morning I launched the dinghy and motored over to Channel Key to bury one more time capsule, took pictures, and made a pirate's map. Then I motored back to *Ka Ching*. She bolted out of the hole like a headstrong mare intent on getting back to the barn—just fifty-five miles to Key West. I arrived at the No. 1 marker at Cow Key Channel at 3:05 p.m., took down the bimini top and antennae, and rumbled down the channel, under Riviera Bridge, and into Riviera Canal like I owned them. Boy, it felt good. Finally, *Ka Ching* executed a nifty 180-degree pirouette into my backyard seawall, and I shut down her engines for the last time. My bride appeared with kisses and hugs. Then, when she was finished with the cats, she gave me a look suggesting that a shower might be nice!

I was so elated with the idea of being home, I celebrated with a fully clothed splash into the pool—and damn-near drowned. I had forgotten that I couldn't raise my head above the water to breathe! But I survived the last hazard, collected some more hugs, and went to bed.

Now it's time for you to up-end a glass with me! You are cordially invited to a docking party at my place this Sunday afternoon, December 12, 2004, from 3:47 p.m. until I fall asleep around 6:32 p.m. (I taught myself a couple of bar tricks you gotta see.) Light bites by Marcia and entertainment by Hope and Faith. No RSVP necessary; just be there!

Love to all.
Gib

Marcia arranged for Teresa, the bartender at all of Dick Moody's parties, to serve at Gib's homecoming celebration. When the party was in full swing, Gib went over to the bar and gestured for everyone to gather round. He indicated that he wanted Teresa to pour his rum and coke into the funnel attached to his PEG tube. Not one to be easily shocked, Teresa said: "Well, this is a first! I have been asked a lot of things in my time, but never to pour booze through a funnel into a guy's stomach!"

On Sunday, January 16, 2005, the *Key West Citizen* told its readers, who had followed Gib's odyssey so avidly through the months, about the completion of the journey.

GIB PETERS' ODYSSEY OF COURAGE BECOMES 'A TALE OF FAITH AND HOPE'
By Joanna Brady Schmida

Many readers who caught the last installment of Gib Peters' diary in this section of the Citizen *several weeks ago have been calling in to inquire about how his trip ended, as he had not yet returned home when writing the last column. He arrived at his house just before Christmas and Marcia Peters was on the seawall before he could swing the boat around in the canal for tie-up, asking a stream of questions her husband could not answer without his computer or his clip board. Now the 68-year-old Peters is back, ready to face the last leg of his journey.*

"I was profoundly affected by the trip," he wrote. "I feel content, fulfilled and blessed."

His serenity stems from coming to terms with his disease in a very personal way, learning as he did to savor every moment and seize every day. Or in Peters' own words, "Up-end the glass. New life is on the way."

When Gib first arrived back home, Faith and Hope, almost full-grown now, hopped off *Ka Ching* to explore the "marina" that was Gib's yard. Inside the house they found something they had never seen before: carpets! This must be paradise! They rolled and clawed and tumbled all over the house. For the first few days after Gib returned home, the cats went back to *Ka Ching* to sleep at night, and he concluded that they had become true sailors. However, after a couple of weeks, as Gib's visits to *Ka Ching* became fewer and he spent more time in the house, they began sleeping curled up with him in his bed.

I saw Gib on December 9 and was shocked at his appearance. He had lost over seventy pounds in the seven months of the trip, but the rate of loss had been greatest in the last few weeks. He was a ghost of his former self. He was unable to hold up his head, and saliva drooled out of his mouth uncontrollably. His arms hung loosely at his sides and flailed around as he walked. He was having some difficulty breathing. It was clear to me that he had starved during the last week of the journey because he did not have the strength to run cans of Jevity Plus into his PEG tube.

I hid my concerns and congratulated him on his truly super-human feat of endurance. I said, "Gib, no one thought you would ever finish the trip, least of all me. I can't tell you how glad I am to have been proven wrong! You are truly a great man. Only some-one as pigheaded as you could have beaten all the odds to do what you've done!"

But it was clear to me that Gib had reached the end of the road, both actually and metaphorically. I talked to him and Marcia about his options. Back when I had first seen him a year and a half earlier, in the summer of 2003, Gib had said that he never wanted to go on a ventilator. By this he meant that he did not want to have a hole made in his windpipe—a tracheotomy—and to be hooked up to a machine that would breathe for him. He had said that in his last days and hours he simply wanted me to keep him comfortable. Now I reminded him about that con-versation and told him that I needed to know if he still felt the same way.

Gib had very little ability to communicate. His arms were paralyzed; he could not speak. However, he clearly mimed that he had not changed his mind on this issue. I asked Marcia if she wanted me to arrange home hospice services for him. Hospice would ensure that, when the end came, he would stay at home and not be taken to the hospital, where they would inevitably put him on a ventilator. At home the hospice doctor and nurses would give him oxygen and medications to let him comfort-ably sleep through the final stages of ALS. However, Marcia was experienced in end-of-life care and insisted upon looking after Gib till the end.

Around this time, Gib learned of the death from cancer of a friend from Shorewood High School. He had sent a letter to him some months earlier and wrote about his difficulty in composing it.

I had the task of writing to a dying friend. It was tough, but I was in the same boat, so I could do it in a candid and direct way. "What does one dying friend say to another dying friend?" I asked. I went on to remind him that we had raised hell together, both had married well and produced four beautiful children each. What more can a man ask for? Then I offered the usual deal. If I got there first, I'd put in a good word for him, if he would do the same for me. I was told he got my letter the day before he died. We connected!

On January 7, 2005, Gib sent me an e-mail saying he knew that he was facing death shortly and did so calmly and with equanimity. He sent me another e-mail on February 3, telling me that he was getting short of breath when lying flat in bed. It was clear that most of the motor neurons supplying his diaphragm and chest muscles had now succumbed to the ALS and he needed a machine to assist his breathing at night. I told him that I would arrange for him to get a non-invasive ventilator, also called a BiPAP machine, and that this did not involve the tracheotomy and permanent ventilator that he feared. I told him that, rather like a CPAP machine used by people with sleep apnea, the BiPAP is usually well tolerated, takes away shortness of breath when lying in bed, and improves quality of life. My nurses arranged for a life support company to visit Gib at home. The respiratory technicians fitted him with the headset and tubes, and the BiPAP machine did help relieve his shortness of breath, making him more comfortable.

Gib spent more and more time in bed. A constant stream of friends came to visit. Everyone could tell that he was failing fast.

Faith and Hope continued to sleep curled up next to Gib, until two days before he died, when they suddenly stopped sleeping on Gib's bed and moved to the other bed in the room, the bed that Marcia had put there for herself.

From: Marcia Peters
To: All of Gib's Friends and Family
Subject: Gib's passing

Gib passed away last night, Saturday, February 26th. He died at home with all of his family at his bedside. Each and every one of you made his last days so rich with your e-mails and encouragement. Thank you for that.

Love to you all!

Marcia

Epilogue

An editorial in the *Key West Citizen* of March 7, 2005, captured what the people of Key West felt about their friend, columnist, and hero, Gib Peters.

> *By any standards, Gib Peters went beyond the concept of ordinary. A devoted husband, a father of four, a successful banker, a trusted adviser and columnist, a generous philanthropist with his professional and personal time, Peters was also an experienced sailor.*
>
> *In May 2004 he set out on a solo voyage that would make him a poet and a seer.*
>
> *Peters' pilgrimage to peace was paced by the progress of his affliction, first diagnosed two years before. ALS is a neurodegenerative disease that left him barely able to write, let alone captain a 29-foot boat for 4,000 miles of Intracoastal Waterway.*
>
> *When he died on February 26, 2005, at the age of 68, Peters had completed 20 dispatches to the* Citizen *about his trip from Key West to New York and back. His story is the most moving expression of life in the face of death that this newspaper has published in generations.*

Gib wished to be cremated. When Marcia went to collect his ashes, she was handed a little casket in a shopping bag with the name of the funeral home on the outside. While driving home with Gib's ashes on the passenger seat beside her, she began talking to him about her sadness at losing him and about what she was planning to do with his ashes. Then she began to wonder what would happen if the police pulled her over and asked her what she was doing. "How can I tell them I'm talking to my husband, who is in a shopping bag on the seat beside me?" She knew it was a moment that would have made Gib chuckle too.

Three days after Gib died, Hope took off and hasn't been seen since. Faith remains at home with Marcia and has become the mascot for her nursing agency.

Gib had requested that his ashes be consigned to the sea that he loved so much. Marcia and Mike had an urn made with a plaque on the side bearing Gib's name and the dates of his birth and death. The family held a celebration of life ceremony in August 2005 and then, accompanied by Mel Fisher's children, they sank the urn among the corals off the Marquesas, exactly where the Spanish treasure ship, *La Nuestra Senora de Atocha*, first struck the reef in 1622. The poem "I'm Free" was read at the ceremony. It epitomizes how Gib wanted people to remember him.

I'm Free

Don't grieve for me, for now I'm free.
I'm following the path God laid for me.
I took His hand when I heard him call,
I turned my back and left it all.

I could not stay another day
To laugh, to love, to work or play.
Tasks left undone must stay that way.
I found that place at the end of the day.

If my parting has left a void,
Then fill it with remembered joy.
A friendship shared, a laugh, a kiss,
Ah yes, these things I too will miss.

Be not burdened with times of sorrow.
I wish you the sunshine of tomorrow.
My life's been full, I savored much.
Good friends, good times, a loved one's touch.

Perhaps my time seemed all too brief,
Don't lengthen it now with undue grief.
Lift up your heart and share with me.
God wanted me now. He set me free.

—Anonymous

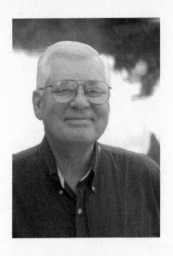

In Memoriam
Gilbert Alexander Peters
April 10, 1936–February 26, 2005

"Up-end the glass! New life is on the way."

Afterword: About ALS

ALS is arguably one of the worst diseases to afflict humans. It is a creeping paralysis that in two years, on average, changes a healthy middle-aged person into a helpless cripple whose every human need has to be provided by a caregiver. He must be lifted in and out of bed, fed, bathed, and cared for like a newborn baby. Though his mind remains perfectly intact, he may eventually become locked into his paralyzed body, unable to speak or move a muscle.

ALS most commonly affects people in their fifties and sixties, though the youngest patient I have seen first developed symptoms at the age of fifteen years. Twenty- and thirty-year-old patients are not uncommon. Men are affected about twice as frequently as women. Though the average survival from onset of symptoms to death is about two years, some patients are dead within three months, while others live more than twenty years.

The disease is confined to the motor system—that is, to the nerve cells that translate our conscious thought to move a limb into nerve impulses that make the muscles move. These motor neurons die in ALS. Sensation, vision, hearing, bladder control, the mind, and memory are all spared. A small number of ALS patients develop a type of mental change called fronto-temporal dementia that affects not memory, as in Alzheimer's disease, but rather judgment and control of behavior.

In the United States, about ten thousand patients develop ALS each year, and about thirty thousand patients are alive with the disease at any point in time. It is often said to be a rare disease, but the number of new cases each year is similar to that of multiple sclerosis. One in 150 deaths among fifty- to seventy-year-olds is due to ALS. To my mind, that is not a rare disease.

A small proportion of patients with ALS, perhaps 10 percent, have relatives with the same disease. We say that they have *familial ALS*. These patients have a mutation of one of their genes, causing the disease; currently we know the genes responsible in about half the families.

Most patients with ALS have no family history. We say they have *sporadic ALS*. At present we do not know what causes the sporadic disease. There must be one or more factors in the environment that cause the disease, and these factors must be present all over the world, since ALS is found everywhere. These environmental factors might be poisons that we are all exposed to, which accumulate in our bodies and in time cause progressive damage to our motor neurons. Presumably most people are able to handle the poisons, to rid them from their bodies, and therefore never develop ALS. Some, though, are unable to stop the poison from killing their motor neurons and wind up developing the disease.

Several regions in the world have an extraordinarily high number of patients with ALS. The island of Guam in the South Pacific and the area around the village of Hohara on the Kii peninsula of Japan are two regions that have one hundred times the amount of ALS that is found in the rest of the world. Research into what causes this high incidence of ALS in Guam—in particular, the brilliant research of Paul Cox and his colleagues at the Institute of EthnoMedicine in Jackson Hole, Wyoming, who are studying links between ALS and a neurotoxin produced by cyanobacteria known as BMAA—is helping us learn the cause of sporadic ALS around the world.

Over the last fifty years, there have been many theories about what causes sporadic ALS. None has so far proved to be correct, and the BMAA theory seems to offer the breakthrough that we have been seeking ever since Jean-Martin Charcot first clearly described ALS in 1874.

Doctors and researchers have tried innumerable drugs to see if they can cure ALS. Many drugs have helped slow the disease in animals with various forms of ALS-type conditions, but most have not worked in human patients with ALS. Currently only one drug, Riluzole, is known to slow the progress of ALS. Gib Peters took Riluzole and also participated in a double-blind placebo-controlled clinical trial of a new drug. That trial meant he had to come back to see me each month. In the end, these visits helped me look after him more closely and keep in contact with the progress of his odyssey. Unfortunately, we found that the new drug Gib was taking did not influence the progression of the disease.

ALS is quite variable in the way that it affects individual patients. In many the disease begins with twitching of the muscles in one limb and slowly develops into weakness and wasting of those muscles. In other patients, there is spasticity, a stiffness and slowness of movement in a limb. For some ALS patients, like Gib Peters, the disease begins in the muscles of speech and swallowing, called bulbar ALS. In most patients the disease slowly spreads to involve all parts of the motor system. Rarely the disease stops and remains unchanged for many years. I have even seen a few patients whose disease has arrested and then gradually improved. Those are the lucky few.

For most ALS sufferers, the disease progresses to the state where they are unable to swallow and may choke on water or food. These patients rapidly lose weight; to maintain their nutrition we have to place a small tube, called a PEG tube, into their stomach through the front of their belly. These patients can then receive full nutrition through the tube and not starve to death—unless, like Gib Peters, they are indulging in extraordinary muscular activity.

Eventually most patients develop respiratory paralysis and will die unless they are put on a respirator and given artificial ventilation. In the United States, when patients are asked to make a choice, most decide not to accept the option of life on a respirator with progressive paralysis. Others make the opposite decision and continue to live happy and productive lives; Stephen Hawking, the renowned astrophysicist, is one such example. Japanese doctors put almost all their ALS patients on respirators, and they frequently live ten or twenty years after they would otherwise have died of respiratory failure. The care of a patient on a respirator is extremely expensive, and in Japan this cost is covered by the government. Few patients in the United States have insurance that is adequate to provide for the cost of life at home on a ventilator, with twenty-four-hour nursing and respiratory care.

Acknowledgments

First and foremost, I want to acknowledge Gib Peters, his wife Marcia, and his children, who gave me so much help in writing this book and so many insights into Gib Peters, the man. I also want to thank every patient with ALS who has allowed me to assist in their care. It is from patients that doctors learn. Doctors are not supposed to let themselves become too friendly with their patients, since it is thought this friendship might cloud their judgment when making difficult decisions. However, doctors, nurses, and health care professionals who care for patients with ALS cannot help but become emotionally attached to them. We have to do so much for our patients and their loved ones. Cry with them when we give them the diagnosis. Provide all the aids and appliances that make continuing function possible. Help them consider a PEG tube or a respirator. Discuss death and how we can prevent suffering in the last few days and hours of life. Mourn with the bereaved family. With all of this, how can we not develop a special friendship with the patient and his family?

Gib and Marcia Peters became my friends. Marcia and her four children lost a beloved husband and father when Gib died of ALS. Their loss was immeasurably greater than mine, but nevertheless I lost a special friend.

Gib did not live long enough to write a book derived from the hilarious yet poignant dispatches he sent while he was on the journey. When approaching death he asked his family to do this for him. This was neither author's narcissism nor a desire for a niche in posterity. He realized that his deep introspection during his time alone on *Ka Ching* had produced something special. What he had learned from facing his own death could be of help to others who are facing the countdown to their own inevitable death.

More than a travelogue, more than the musings of a dying man, *Gib's Odyssey—A Tale of Faith and Hope on the Intracoastal Waterway* is a tale of the triumph of the human spirit, an insight into the unfathomable cycle of birth, life, death, and new birth. When Gib was expecting his first grandchild, his first glimpse of that cycle prompted him to compose the toast that ended each of his e-mails: "Up-end the glass! New life is on the way."

Marcia, her children, and I searched long and hard for someone with more skill than I to compose Gib's stories into a book. I had promised Gib that if no one else would write it then I would take on the task. In some ways I look on this book as my last contribution to Gib's care—the last thing that I as his doctor could do for him. I feel guilty that he died. I continue to be distressed that after spending forty years caring for patients with ALS and doing research to find the cause of the disease, I still have no effective way to treat it. This book is, in part, an attempt to tell the world more about ALS so that more research can be done to find the cause and eventual cure of the disease.

Gib would have understood that the completion of this book is for me both an apology for that failure and a statement of hope. It is my small way to ensure that he has not shuffled off this mortal coil without leaving his mark. And, as I said to Gib when I first told him that he had ALS: "One day, I will be able to sit here and tell you that you have ALS, but not to worry; we have a way to cure it!" It's a hope I still carry for a day that can't come soon enough.

In the process of researching and writing the book, I have been helped by too many people for me to name them all. My thanks are due especially to the members of Gib Peters's immediate family: Marcia, Mike, Lisa, Kim, and Lynnea and George Cruse. I'm also grateful to Gib Peters' close friends—Madeleine Burnside, Walton Dutcher Jr., Caroline and Jerry Cash, Bobby Highsmith, Phil Miani, Dick and Kathleen Moody, and Bill Schwessinger— and to the staff of the *Key West Citizen*. I particularly want to thank Louis Berney and several other friends who read the manuscript at various stages of preparation. Special thanks go to my literary agent, Albert LaFarge, and Janice Goldklang, publisher at Globe Pequot Press, for their great help in editing the final manuscript.

Last but not least, I want to thank my wonderful wife, Jeanne Baker, for her unfailing support and insight as we go together through the voyage of life, and my five children for being the terrific people they are.

Walter G. Bradley, DM, FRCP
Miami, March 2010

About the Author

Walter G. Bradley, DM, FRCP, is the emeritus chairman of the Department of Neurology at the Miller School of Medicine, University of Miami. A 1963 graduate of the medical school at Oxford University, Dr. Bradley has cared for patients with ALS and done research to find the cause and cure of the condition for more than forty years. In 2006 he received the prestigious Forbes Norris Award of the International Alliance of ALS/MND Associations.

In addition to serving as lead editor of the best-selling textbook of neurology, *Neurology in Clinical Practice,* Dr. Bradley has written more than two hundred peer-reviewed articles, more than one hundred chapters and reviews, and several online publications on health care reform. He is also the author of nearly thirty books, including, most recently, *Treating the Brain: What the Best Doctors Know.*

Dr. Bradley has five grown children, three sons and two daughters. He lives with his wife, Jeanne Baker, Esq., near Miami, Florida.